100 Questions & Answers About Hip Replacement

Stuart J. Fischer, MD
Summit Orthopaedics and Sports Medicine,
Summit, NJ

JONES AND BARTLETT PUBLISHERS

Sudbury, Massachusetts

BOSTON   TORONTO   LONDON   SINGAPORE

World Headquarters

Jones and Bartlett Publishers
40 Tall Pine Drive
Sudbury, MA 01776
978-443-5000
info@jbpub.com
www.jbpub.com

Jones and Bartlett Publishers
Canada
6339 Ormindale Way
Mississauga, Ontario L5V 1J2
Canada

Jones and Bartlett Publishers
International
Barb House, Barb Mews
London W6 7PA
United Kingdom

Jones and Bartlett's books and products are available through most bookstores and online booksellers. To contact Jones and Bartlett Publishers directly, call 800-832-0034, fax 978-443-8000, or visit our website, www.jbpub.com.

Substantial discounts on bulk quantities of Jones and Bartlett's publications are available to corporations, professional associations, and other qualified organizations. For details and specific discount information, contact the special sales department at Jones and Bartlett via the above contact information or send an email to specialsales@jbpub.com.

The authors, editor, and publisher have made every effort to provide accurate information. However, they are not responsible for errors, omissions, or for any outcomes related to the use of the contents of this book and take no responsibility for the use of the products and procedures described. Treatments and side effects described in this book may not be applicable to all people; likewise, some people may require a dose or experience a side effect that is not described herein. Drugs and medical devices are discussed that may have limited availability controlled by the Food and Drug Administration (FDA) for use only in a research study or clinical trial. Research, clinical practice, and government regulations often change the accepted standard in this field. When consideration is being given to use of any drug in the clinical setting, the healthcare provider or reader is responsible for determining FDA status of the drug, reading the package insert, and reviewing prescribing information for the most up-to-date recommendations on dose, precautions, and contraindications, and determining the appropriate usage for the product. This is especially important in the case of drugs that are new or seldom used.

Production Credits

Executive Publisher: Christopher Davis
Editorial Assistant: Sara Cameron
Associate Production Editor: Leah Corrigan
Senior Marketing Manager: Barb Bartoszek
Manufacturing and Inventory Supervisor:
   Amy Bacus

Cover Designer: Carolyn Downer
Cover Images: © Photodisc, © American
   Academy of Orthopaedic Surgeons,
   © Photodisc
Printing and Binding: Malloy, Inc.
Cover Printing: Malloy, Inc.

Library of Congress Cataloging-in-Publication Data
Fischer, Stuart J.
   100 questions and answers about hip replacement / Stuart J. Fischer.
      p. cm. — (100 questions & answers)
   ISBN 978-0-7637-6872-0 (alk. paper)
   1. Total hip replacement—Surgery—Popular works. 2. Hip joint—Surgery—Popular works. I. Title. II. Title: One hundred questions and answers about hip replacement.
   RD549.F57 2011
   617.5'810592—dc22

                                                                2009050532

6048

Printed in the United States of America
14 13 12 11 10   10 9 8 7 6 5 4 3 2 1

To my wife Doreen and my children Anna, Sara, and Lisa

and

To my mother Charlotte Fischer, and my father Dr. Leo Fischer,
the first orthopaedic surgeon in the family.

Contents

Acknowledgments   ix

Part 1: Introduction   1

Questions 1–3 introduce readers to some basic facts about hip replacements:
- What is a hip replacement?
- Why should I have a hip replacement?
- When were the first total hip replacements done? How many are done each year?

Part 2: Hip Disease   9

Questions 4–11 discuss the anatomy of the hip and the different medical conditions that can affect the hip, such as:
- What are the parts of a normal hip joint?
- What is *osteoarthritis*?
- What is arthritis secondary to childhood hip disease?

Part 3: Symptoms   29

Questions 12–16 review common symptoms associated with hip problems:
- Why does my hip hurt? Where does it hurt?
- Why do I limp? Why does my leg feel short?
- Why does my hip sometimes make a crackling noise when I try to move it?

Part 4: Diagnosis   35

Questions 17–22 explain how medical conditions relating to the hip are diagnosed, such as:
- How will my doctor make the diagnosis of an arthritic hip?
- Do I need an MRI?
- What is an arthrogram? When is it done?

Part 5: Treatment without Surgery 51

Questions 23–28 discuss nonsurgical options available in treating an injured hip:
- Will it help to lose weight?
- What are NSAIDs?
- Do supplements like Glucosamine help?

Part 6: Surgery 61

Questions 29–36 review the types of surgery common in hip replacement:
- Can I have a total hip replacement if I have had previous hip surgery?
- What is Bipolar (Partial) Hip Replacement?
- What is resurfacing?

Part 7: The Operation—Total Hip Replacement 89

Questions 37–50 offer tips on how to prepare for and what to expect with hip replacement surgery:
- How can I prepare for surgery?
- Who will do the surgery?
- How is the surgery done?

Part 8: After Surgery 125

Questions 51–67 review the steps taken by you and your doctors after hip replacement surgery is performed:
- What kind of medication will I be given for pain?
- What precautions do I need to take against dislocation?
- What kind of physical therapy will I need?

Part 9: Risks and Complications 155

Questions 68–80 explore the risks that may arise during or after the surgery and how to best manage any complications, such as:
- How do I know if I have an infection? How can an infection be diagnosed?
- What is a dislocation? What can cause dislocation?
- What other medical complications can happen from surgery?

Part 10: Revisions and Fractures 189

Questions 81–89 explain how previously replaced hips can sustain damage and how these issues are rectified:
- When is revision surgery necessary?
- How do I know if my hip has loosened?
- Are there greater risks from revision surgery?

Part 11: Other Questions 213

Contents

Questions 90–100 offer answers to other common inquiries about life before, during, and after hip replacement surgery:

- What can my family do to help?
- Can both hips be replaced at the same time?
- Can I get pregnant if I have had a total hip replacement?

Glossary 235

Index 243

Acknowledgments

Great things happen when you work with great people. I am indebted to many for their help and advice in preparing this book and in practicing orthopaedic surgery for thirty years.

With this in mind, I would like to express my thanks to:

The staff of the American Academy of Orthopaedic Surgeons in Rosemont, Illinois:

- Marilyn Fox, Jane Baque, Laura Giblin (Publications)
- Sandy Gordon (Public Relations)
- Mark Wieting and Jeff Kramer (Education)
- Mary Ann Porucznik (AAOS Now)

Bev Lynch, Pam Passman, and Lauren Myers. They have made the New Jersey Orthopaedic Society one of the most successful state medical organizations in the country. Their help in running the organization and building the OSNJ Medical Liability Purchasing Alliance has been invaluable.

The editors, committee members, and council chairs I have worked with at the American Academy of Orthopaedic Surgeons.

The faculty at New York Orthopaedic Hospital, including my chairmen, Drs. Frank Stinchfield and Alexander Garcia. Dr. Stinchfield, one of the pioneers of hip surgery in the United States, taught me how to do a total hip. Dr. Garcia asked me to write my first review article on hip surgery.

My wonderful staff who do everything for me and make my practice run smoothly:

- Lucy
- Tracy (who compiled the glossary for this book)
- Vicky
- Yolanda

- Beverly
- Barbara
- Pat
- Sheena
- Sandra

Lana Karasina, my operating room nurse and first assistant for the past twelve years. She assists on all my total hips. Lana knows what instruments I need before I need them.

Carmine Battinelli, my technologist and assistant for twenty-five years. Carmine is a superb x-ray technician and is loved both by patients and everyone around him. He is simply the best there is.

Dawn and her staff at The Center For Ambulatory Surgery in Mountainside, New Jersey, who take such great care of my patients.

The operating room team at Overlook Hospital in Summit, New Jersey, where I have been doing hip replacement surgery since I started practice.

The orthopaedic nurses and therapists at Overlook Hospital who guide my hip patients from preoperative classes through rehabilitation after surgery.

My orthopaedic colleagues at The Center For Ambulatory Surgery, Overlook Hospital, and the New Jersey Orthopaedic Society.

Dr. Stuart Hirsch, my friend and orthopaedic mentor. Stuart helped me go over text and pictures for this book. He has been a leader at both the state and national levels. No one has done more to make orthopaedic surgery better for both doctors and patients in New Jersey than Stuart.

And of course my family who have been so patient and understanding during the many long nights and weekends I have spent putting together this book.

PART ONE

Introduction

What is a hip replacement?

Why should I have a hip replacement?

When were the first total hip replacements done?
How many are done each year?

More . . .

1. What is a hip replacement?

A hip replacement is the removal of all or part of the hip joint and insertion of an artificial ball or an artificial ball and socket. The diseased bone and joint surfaces are replaced with new or prosthetic parts.

The new parts are called *components* or *implants*. They are called implants because they are inserted or implanted in a patient's body.

A hip replacement may be partial or total. In a **total hip replacement**, both the ball of the hip joint

Total hip replacement

A hip joint replacement where both the ball of the hip joint (femoral head) and the hip joint socket (acetabulum) are removed and replaced with artificial or prosthetic parts.

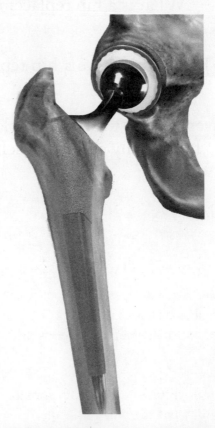

Figure 1   Illustration of total hip replacement components.

Courtesy of Smith and Nephew.

(**femoral head**) and the hip joint socket (**acetabulum**) are removed and replaced. In a partial replacement, only the femur is replaced and the socket is left intact.

Femoral head

The round part or ball of the hip joint.

Acetabulum

Socket of the hip joint.

In the 40 years since hip replacements were first performed, millions of people around the world have experienced relief from disabling hip disease. They have been able to walk and to resume normal function pain free. Total hip replacement has been considered a modern medical miracle.

This book is a guide to the many facets of hip replacement surgery. It is meant to provide information about hips, hip disease, and hip surgery that is detailed but coherent and easy to read. In addition, this book will:

- Tell you about the different kinds of hip replacements.
- Explain why you might be a candidate for surgery.
- Review the anatomy of a normal hip.
- Show you what happens when your hip stops functioning normally.
- Review the causes of hip pain and hip disease.
- Describe the symptoms of a bad hip.
- Tell you how your doctor makes the diagnosis of an arthritic hip.
- Outline the nonsurgical treatment of hip disease.
- Discuss the surgical options for different types of hip disease and different patients.
- Tell you about orthopaedic surgeons and what they do.
- Explain how the procedure is done.
- Describe the different types of implants that are available and what they are made of.
- Tell you what to expect during your hospital stay and afterward.

- Outline the physical therapy and rehabilitation you will need after surgery.
- Talk about the care of your new hip joint.
- List the risks of surgery and their consequences.
- Discuss procedures that can be done instead of hip replacement to treat a painful hip.

The book will also tell you what happens when you need to have a second or *revision* surgery on the same hip. It will review some of the many advances in hip replacement technology.

Most important, the one hundred questions and answers will encourage you to seek new information. As you read through the book, try to think of the questions you need to ask your doctor and other things you want to know about this very successful operation.

2. Why should I have a hip replacement?

The main reason to have a hip replacement is relief of pain. When your hip joint is damaged or diseased it can be severely painful. Along with the pain, you can lose motion in your hip and have difficulty walking. It becomes harder to perform your routine activities. In short, your diseased or damaged hip interferes with the quality of your day-to-day life.

A painful hip can affect other parts of your body. You may develop back pain as you try to compensate for loss of motion in your hip. You may feel pain in your knee or in your opposite leg as you try to relieve pressure on your bad side. If your mobility is limited, you may gain weight because you are unable to exercise.

Hip replacement can relieve pain and improve the strength and motion in your hip. In some cases the results are dramatic. Many patients note that even a day or two after the procedure they have pain in their incision, but the joint pain they had before surgery is largely gone.

For most people, hip replacement surgery is *elective*. It is done for conditions such as osteoarthritis, which are not life threatening but affect your life in other ways. It is a procedure that is planned and scheduled ahead of time. It is not something you have to do, but is something you choose to do. Unlike an appendectomy, it is not an emergency procedure. The decision to have a hip replacement is made after consultation with an orthopaedic surgeon, but ultimately, the decision is yours.

For a few patients, hip replacement has to be done on an urgent basis. If a hip is broken (**fractured**), surgery should be done as soon as possible to relieve pain and allow the patient to get out of bed. Hip replacement is the treatment of choice for some fractures. Bone tumors in the hip also require urgent treatment because the tumor will continue to grow and cause further damage to the bone.

Fracture
A crack or break in a bone.

There is more to hip replacement than just the surgical procedure. There is preoperative planning, testing, and medical evaluation. After surgery there is time in the hospital, therapy, and rehabilitation. And of course life is different with an artificial joint in your body.

As you consider surgery, take time to learn about your hip, what treatment is available and why you would be a candidate for hip replacement.

Margaret K., a patient, says:

My new hip felt perfectly natural and totally pain free.

3. When were the first total hip replacements done? How many are done each year?

Hip replacement surgery has been a work in progress for more than 80 years. Dr. Marius Smith-Petersen in Boston developed the *cup arthroplasty* in the 1920s and 1930s. Damaged bone from the hip joint was removed and a metal cup was placed over the head of the femur. While this wasn't truly a replacement, it was an attempt to put new surfaces in a damaged joint. The cup arthroplasty remained the primary surgical treatment for an arthritic hip for 25 years.

Partial hip replacement

A hip joint replacement where only the femur is replaced with an artificial or prosthetic part. The hip joint socket (acetabulum) is left intact.

The first **partial hip replacement** was performed by Dr. Austin Moore at Johns Hopkins University in the early 1940s. Only the femoral head was replaced, not the socket. It consisted of a large metal ball with a stem that fit inside the **shaft** of the femur. The Austin Moore **prosthesis** was modified in the 1950s and became the standard treatment for certain types of hip fractures.

Shaft

The long portion of a bone. In the femur it is the segment between the hip and the knee.

Prosthesis

An artificial component or implant used to replace a damaged or diseased body part.

The modern total hip replacement was pioneered by Sir John Charnley at Wrightington, England in 1962. For this surgery, a small metal ball and stem that fit inside a plastic or **polyethylene** socket were used. Both components were inserted in bone and held in place with bone cement. The femoral head was smaller than normal so as to create less friction and wear in the socket. Dr. Charnley called his procedure "low friction arthroplasty." Even though cement is now used less frequently, the concept of a metal femoral head articulating with a polyethylene socket remains the gold standard in hip replacement to this day.

Polyethylene

A strong plastic material used as the bearing surface in most acetabular components.

In the United States, more than half a million hip replacement procedures are done annually. According to data from the Department of Health and Human Services National Hospital Discharge Survey, 231,000 total and 251,000 partial hip replacements were performed in the United States in 2006. An additional 38,000 revision procedures were done on hips that had previous surgery. This represented an increase of more than 200,000 surgeries in an 8-year period.

As our population ages and medical advances help people to live longer it is expected that the number of hip replacements done annually will continue to grow.

PART TWO

Hip Disease

What are the parts of a normal hip joint?

What is *osteoarthritis*?

What is arthritis secondary to childhood hip disease?

More . . .

4. What are the parts of a normal hip joint?

A joint is a structure in the body, made up of two or more bones, that allows one bone to move against another. Movement through joints lets different parts of the body change positions.

The hip is a ball and socket joint. Unlike a hinge joint, a ball and socket has multiple planes of movement. The socket is called the *acetabulum*. It is made up of portions of three bones—the ilium, the ischium, and the pubis.

The femur is a single specific bone. At the hip joint, it is divided into several anatomic areas. The round part, or the ball, is called the *femoral head*. The section below the ball is called the **femoral neck**. There are two bony

Femoral neck

The section of bone in the hip joint below the femoral head (or ball).

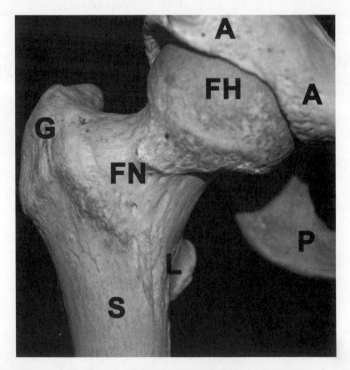

Figure 2 Model of a normal hip joint showing: (A) acetabulum or socket, (FH) femoral head, (FN) femoral neck, (G) greater trochanter, (L) lesser trochanter, (P) pelvis, and (S) shaft or long portion of femur.

prominences below the femoral neck. The outer prominence, the **greater trochanter**, is the large bony surface that you can feel on the outside of your hip. The abductor muscles, that pull your leg outward, attach to the greater trochanter. A smaller bump on the inside of the hip is called the **lesser trochanter**. This is where the main muscle that flexes the hip, the *iliopsoas*, attaches.

The region between the greater and lesser trochanters is called **intertrochanteric**. The part of the femur below the two trochanters is called **subtrochanteric**. The bone on the inner side of the femoral neck is called the **calcar**. The shaft of the femur is the long portion of the bone between the hip and the knee joints.

Several soft tissue structures are present around and within the hip joint. The lining of the hip joint is called the **capsule**. The back or posterior portion of the capsule supplies a large part of the blood supply to the head of the femur. The *labrum* is a ring of thick tissue called *fibrocartilage* around the edge of the socket. It adds depth to the socket and stability to the hip. The **ligamentum teres** is a thick ligament that extends from a portion of the acetabulum called **acetabular notch** to an area of the femur called the **fovea**. It carries a small portion of the blood supply to the femoral head.

Within the joint is a lining tissue called **synovium**. Synovial tissue is found in every large joint in the body. It secretes synovial fluid, which lubricates and nourishes the tissues inside the joint.

The surfaces of the joint are made up of smooth white tissue called **articular cartilage**. It is damage to the cartilage surfaces of the joint that usually creates the need for hip replacement surgery.

Greater trochanter

Bony prominence located below the femoral neck of the hip where muscles attach that abduct the hip.

Lesser trochanter

Small bony prominence below the femoral neck of the femur where the iliopsoas muscle attaches.

Intertrochanteric

Area of the femur below the femoral neck between the greater and lesser trochanters.

Subtrochanteric

Part of the femur below the two trochanters.

Calcar

The bone on the inner side of the neck of the femur.

Capsule

The lining tissue that surrounds the hip joint.

Ligamentum teres

A thick ligament that extends from an area of the acetabulum called the acetabular notch to a point on the femur called the fovea. It carries a portion of the blood supply to the femoral head.

Acetabular notch

A small recess inside the acetabulum where the ligamentum teres inserts.

Fovea

A notch on the surface of the femoral head where blood vessels enter.

Synovium

Lining tissue inside a joint which secretes synovial fluid to lubricate and nourish the joint.

Articular cartilage

The smooth, white tissue that covers the surfaces of a joint. (see also Hyaline Cartilage)

Together all the parts of the joint combine to form a strong stable structure that allows for friction-free movement in many directions.

5. What happens when my hip joint doesn't work normally?

The process of degeneration, or breakdown, of a hip joint is a gradual one but may proceed at different speeds depending upon the cause. When one part of the hip is affected by disease or injury, it can affect the function of the entire joint.

The part most often affected is the articular cartilage. In a healthy joint, the friction between two moving surfaces is less than between two ice cubes sliding against one another. When the cartilage is damaged or starts to wear down, the joint can no longer move smoothly.

A defect in the surface of the articular cartilage will wear against the opposite side of the joint and cause damage to that area as well. The joint surfaces collapse and the underlying bone is affected. It may become deformed. The joint loses range of motion and weight bearing forces in the joint are altered.

At the same time, the lining tissues within the joint become inflamed. The soft tissues around the joint such as the joint capsule may become tightened and contracted. The muscles that move the joint may become weakened. When all this happens, the hip joint can no longer function normally.

Many disease processes can damage the hip joint. Most are related to some form of arthritis. They will be discussed in detail in the next few chapters.

There are five major causes of hip disease:

- Osteoarthritis
- Rheumatoid arthritis
- Post-traumatic arthritis
- Avascular necrosis
- Arthritis secondary to childhood hip disease

Some of the secondary less common causes include:

- Prior infection
- Hemophilia
- Ankylosing spondylitis
- Gaucher's disease
- Sickle cell anemia
- Paget's disease

Each of these conditions is different in how it changes the anatomy and biology of the normal hip joint. All of them can create the need for hip replacement.

6. *What is* osteoarthritis?

Osteoarthritis is the most common diagnosis for patients having total hip replacement. It is also the most common type of arthritis. The vast majority of all patients, men and women, undergoing hip replacement have osteoarthritis.

Osteoarthritis is arthritis due to age, repetitive activity, or simple everyday wear and tear. It affects only one joint or a few joints in the body at one time. It is not a systemic process like rheumatoid arthritis. It affects only joints, not other organs in the body.

More than 30 million people in the United States are estimated to have osteoarthritis. Symptoms may develop

Osteoarthritis is the most common diagnosis for patients having total hip replacement.

at any time, usually after age 40 years, and the incidence increases with age. It is more common in women. As the population becomes older more people will develop the disease.

No one knows what triggers the onset of osteoarthritis. Besides age and overuse, other factors include being overweight, joint laxity, joint deformity, and abnormal articular cartilage. Long-term high impact activities such as sports can also cause damage to the joint surfaces.

The hips, knees, hands, neck, and lower back are the areas most affected by osteoarthritis. It is estimated that by age 65 half of the population has x-ray changes of osteoarthritis in at least one joint. A smaller percentage, however, are actually symptomatic. Symptoms do not always correlate directly with the amount of damage seen on x-ray. You may have severe pain even though an x-ray shows only mild damage to the joint.

Sclerotic

Hard dense bone that forms beneath the surface in an arthritic joint.

Spurs

Bony prominences that form at the edges of an arthritic joint. (see also Osteophytes)

The main cause of osteoarthritis is breakdown of the joint surface, the articular cartilage. As the body gets older the cartilage loses its elasticity. It can no longer absorb shock and compressive forces as it once did. It loses the ability to repair itself. When this happens, the joint surface starts to collapse. The underlying bone called *subchondral bone* reacts by becoming hard or **sclerotic**. It has a dense or thick white look on x-ray. Bone cysts called *subchondral cysts* may form in this location. The bone becomes deformed and forms prominences called **spurs** or **osteophytes** at the edges of the joint.

When the joint cartilage has completely worn away an x-ray will show *bone on bone*. One bone in the joint can be seen rubbing up against another with no joint space left in between.

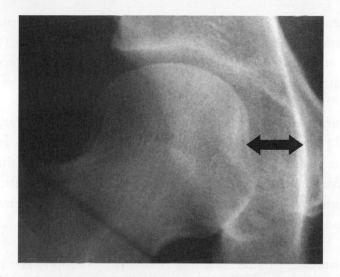

Figure 3   X-ray of a normal hip joint. The femoral head is round. Arrows indicate a normal joint space between the head of the femur and the acetabulum.

© American Academy of Orthopaedic Surgeons.

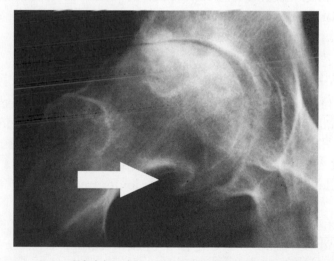

Figure 4   X-ray of hip joint with osteoarthritis. The femoral head is no longer round and the joint space is narrow. Arrow points to the large spur at the edge of the femoral head.

Pain is the main symptom of an arthritic joint. Stiffness, loss of motion, and weakness develop as the disease gets worse. The progress of the disease varies among individuals and even from joint to joint in the same person. Some people may go along for years with the same level of pain and no x-ray changes. Others have complete destruction of a joint and need surgery within a few short months.

Surgery is indicated when you can no longer tolerate the pain and limitation caused by an arthritic joint. In the hip, total hip replacement or **arthroplasty** is the procedure most often performed for osteoarthritis. Other procedures such as **resurfacing**, fusion, **osteotomy**, and **arthroscopy** will be discussed later in this book.

Osteoarthritis is not osteoporosis. Osteoporosis is thinning of the bones in your body. Like osteoarthritis it comes on as the body ages. Unlike osteoarthritis it does not directly involve joints. You can have weak thin bone and still have normal joints. Osteoporosis can predispose to fractures but it is not painful. It is completely different from osteoarthritis.

7. *What is* rheumatoid arthritis?

Rheumatoid arthritis is a systemic disease that affects multiple joints in the body. Unlike osteoarthritis, which is due to age and wear, rheumatoid arthritis is the result of a disease process throughout the entire body. As a rule, multiple rather than single joints are affected.

Rheumatoid arthritis usually develops between ages 30 and 60 years, but can also present earlier as *juvenile arthritis* in childhood. Women are more than twice as likely to have the disease as men. There may be a genetic predisposition to getting the disease. Some evidence suggests that rheumatoid arthritis may be an autoimmune phenomenon, but it is unclear as to what triggers the immune response.

Arthroplasty

A procedure performed to reconstruct a diseased or deformed joint. It is commonly used to refer to joint replacement surgery.

Resurfacing

A type of hip replacement that preserves the femoral neck and inner portion of the femoral head. Only the articular cartilage and outer portion of the femoral head are removed.

Osteotomy

An operation where a section of the bone is cut so that the bone may be realigned to a better position.

Arthroscopy

A surgical technique where surgery on a joint is performed through tiny incisions with a fiberoptic scope, small instruments and a video camera.

The source of the disease is the *synovium*, the lining tissue of the joint. In a healthy joint, synovium provides lubrication and nutrition to the surrounding tissues. In rheumatoid arthritis, the synovium becomes inflamed and proliferates. The resulting tissue layer is called **pannus**. Pannus invades the joint surfaces and causes destruction of the cartilage and underlying bone. Inflammatory factors in the synovial fluid may also damage the cartilage.

Pannus

Inflamed synovial tissue in a joint with rheumatoid arthritis that invades and destroys joint surfaces.

The diagnosis of rheumatoid arthritis is based largely on clinical factors, but blood tests may also be positive. The *rheumatoid factor*, an antibody found in blood, is present in most patients with rheumatoid arthritis. The *erythrocyte sedimentation rate (ESR)* is a less specific test that is often elevated in RA.

The American College of Rheumatology lists seven criteria for the diagnosis of rheumatoid arthritis. Four of these have to be positive in order to confirm the diagnosis. The seven criteria include:

- Morning stiffness
- Arthritis in at lease three joints
- Arthritis in the hands
- Joint involvement on both sides of the body
- Positive rheumatoid factor
- Rheumatoid nodules
- X-ray changes consistent with rheumatoid arthritis

Joints with rheumatoid arthritis are warm, swollen, and sometimes contracted. Other clinical features include rheumatoid nodules beneath the skin and *tenosynovitis* or thickening of the tissue that covers tendons.

The hip is one of many joints in the body that can be affected by RA. Like OA, the onset is gradual. The main symptoms are pain, stiffness, loss of motion, and limping. Usually the diagnosis of rheumatoid arthritis is known to the patient by the time symptoms present in the hip.

The surgical treatment for RA is the same as for OA. If the joint is destroyed total hip replacement is required.

Rheumatoid bone is often osteoporotic and of poor quality. This may affect the choice of components and the type of fixation. If the bone is very soft it may not be possible to press fit components and cement may be required. Patients with rheumatoid arthritis are not candidates for resurfacing because of the risk of bone collapse and failure.

8. *What is* post-traumatic arthritis?

Post-traumatic arthritis is arthritis of the hip joint that develops after an injury.

Post-traumatic arthritis is arthritis of the hip joint that develops after an injury. The injury can be a severe contusion to the hip or a fracture of one of the bones within or near the joint.

A hard bruise to the hip joint or fall on the hip may not always cause a visible fracture in bone. It can, however, cause an injury to the surface or articular cartilage of the joint. The damaged surface no longer moves smoothly and the joint deteriorates and develops arthritis.

Articular injuries are hard to diagnose because the joint surfaces cannot be seen on plain x-ray. Injuries to the joint may sometimes be diagnosed on MRI. Other times, the joint injury can present as prolonged pain and stiffness with no positive radiologic findings at all. Months or years later, arthritis can develop and the severity of the joint injury is evident.

Most often post-traumatic arthritis develops after a fracture in or around the hip. Fractures through the head of the femur are unusual but can occur either as an isolated injury or in combination with a **dislocation**. Fractures into the hip joint socket, the acetabulum, are more common. Either of these injuries results in a damaged joint surface and can lead to post-traumatic arthritis.

Arthritis can also result from fractures that do not directly involve the joint. Examples are an intertrochanteric fracture of the hip or a fracture of the long portion or shaft of the femur. Even though the fracture heals away from the joint, the shape of the femur may change and this can lead to altered mechanics in the joint. Some parts of the joint may develop abnormal pressure and subsequent arthritis.

Since it results from injury, post traumatic arthritis is most often unilateral or involves one hip only. Injuries to both hips are less common. They usually result from high velocity trauma such as an automobile accident.

Post-traumatic arthritis can develop following a low impact osteoporotic fracture in the elderly. The incidence is lower in these fractures because elderly people place less demand on their hips and have a shorter life span in which to develop the arthritic symptoms.

Hip replacement in post-traumatic arthritis is different than a routine primary total hip. If there has been previous surgery, there may be hardware which needs to be removed. Scar tissue may be present which makes dissection more difficult. A fracture deformity of the femur may make it harder to place standard components. A defect in the acetabulum may require a bone graft.

In general, the symptoms of post-traumatic arthritis are similar to osteoarthritis, but the surgery can sometimes be a little more difficult.

Dislocation
When the ball of the hip joint comes out of the socket.

9. *What is* avascular necrosis?

Avascular necrosis (AVN) or **osteonecrosis** is a disease where the blood flow to the femoral head is damaged. Part of the bone of the femoral head then undergoes *necrosis*—it dies. When the bone dies, it becomes painful. The pain may be present either with activity or at rest. The joint surface of the femoral head may collapse and arthritis will result.

Symptoms usually present twelve to eighteen months after the initial damage to the bone. The causes of AVN may be traumatic such as dislocation or femoral neck fracture, or may be atraumatic and systemic.

When the cause is traumatic, a fracture disrupts the blood supply to the femoral head. Blood vessels run

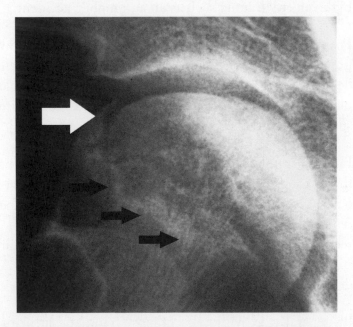

Figure 5   X-ray of femoral head with avascular necrosis. The joint surface of the femur has collapsed and fractured (white arrow). The fracture line extends into the femoral head (black arrows).

through the posterior capsule of the hip joint which is injured by the fracture. The blood supply to the femoral head is interrupted and AVN develops. A similar mechanism happens with traumatic dislocation. The head of the femur is forced out of the socket and the capsule is torn. Most often dislocation occurs in a posterior direction.

Some studies show that the time from when the hip is dislocated to when it is put back in place is a factor in whether AVN develops. The shorter the time the better. AVN may develop following a femoral neck fracture even though the fracture itself heals.

Many systemic factors have been felt to lead to avascular necrosis. These include:

- Steroid therapy
- Alcoholism
- Collagen vascular disease
- Gaucher's disease
- Arterial occlusion
- Blood clotting disorders
- Other diseases of circulation
- Other blood diseases called *hemoglobinopathies* where small vessels in the head of the femur may be occluded.

Radiation injury and *caisson*, or dysbaric disease, are two other causes of AVN which do not fit the trauma or systemic categories. Radiation injury follows large doses of radiation given to a patient to treat other conditions. **Caisson disease** can occur in deep sea divers who return to the surface too quickly without allowing adequate time to decompress. With good training this rarely happens.

Caisson disease

A disease that can cause avascular necrosis. It occurs in deep sea divers who return to the surface too quickly without allowing adequate time to decompress.

Patients who have had organ transplants are known to develop avascular necrosis, possibly because they take medication to suppress their immune systems. In some cases, the cause of AVN may be **idiopathic**. This means that it develops spontaneously with no known cause.

Idiopathic
Condition that develops sponta- neously with no known cause.

Even though steroid therapy is one of the most common causes of AVN it is not known what dose of steroids or what length of treatment causes the disease. In systemic conditions, it is not clear if AVN occurs with a single insult to the circulation or gradually over time. It may be the result of multiple insults to the bone marrow in the same area.

The first symptom of avascular necrosis is pain. At the onset of the disease, the hip maintains a good range of motion. As the disease progresses, range of motion decreases. Examination and x-ray findings become similar to those in osteoarthritis. AVN is different from osteoarthritis, however, because disease first develops in the bone rather than in the joint.

AVN is differ- ent from osteoarthritis, however, because disease first develops in the bone rather than in the joint.

On x-ray, AVN appears as a wedge of abnormal bone in the superior, or upper, part of the head of the femur. On a lateral x-ray a *crescent sign* may be visible. This is a clear line just below the surface of the joint. At this point the surface remains intact and has not collapsed. Within the femoral head an area of dense whitish appearing bone is visible. This indicates a process of bone repair called *creeping substitution*.

Often the diagnosis and surgical treatment of AVN are delayed. If pain is present and there are no changes on x-ray, the diagnosis may sometimes be made with an MRI study. Patients may delay treatment until symptoms are more severe. At the very least they should seek an orthopaedic consultation. If they wait too long, some of the more conservative options such as **core decompression** may no longer be helpful and hip replacement is required.

Hip replacement is not the only treatment option for avascular necrosis. If the disease is not far advanced, then other procedures may be done in an attempt to save the femoral head. This is particularly true for patients in their 30s and 40s. More conservative procedures include:

- Core decompression with or without bone grafting
- Bone grafting through a cortical window
- Osteotomy
- Resurfacing

Resurfacing may not be possible if there is too much bone collapse or there is involvement of the bone in the neck of the femur.

For older patients and for younger patients in whom the femoral head has collapsed, hip replacement is the surgical treatment of choice.

10. What is arthritis secondary to childhood hip disease?

There are three major types of childhood hip problems that can lead to arthritis in adult years:

- Developmental dysplasia of the hip (DDH)
- Perthes disease
- Slipped capital femoral epiphysis (SCFE)

Each of these diseases develops early on in life. DDH is present at birth and is usually diagnosed at that time or

Core decompression

A surgical procedure to treat avascular necrosis done by drilling the femoral neck and femoral head.

within the first year of life. Perthes disease presents as hip pain or a limp between ages 3 and 8 years. Slipped capital femoral epiphysis occurs in young adolescents between ages 11 and 14 years. All of these diseases may be treated successfully during childhood years but may then cause symptomatic arthritis later on. After treatment, patients may have normal function with little or no pain until early adult years or middle age. Some may have a limp or a residual rotation of the leg. Most patients, however, are active and participate in sports and athletic activities well into their adult years.

As with other forms of arthritis, the time to consider surgery is when you can no longer tolerate the pain. Disease may be unilateral or bilateral if both hips were affected by the disease. Surgery in these situations may

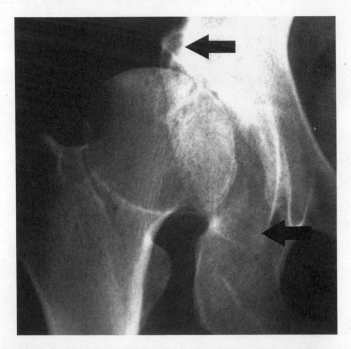

Figure 6 DDH. The femoral head and neck are deformed. The socket (arrows) is long flat and vertical.

be more complicated because of the residual anatomic deformity.

In DDH, the hip joint socket may be relatively high and shallow. The hip may be dislocated and form a false socket above the normal anatomic level. The femoral canal may be small and narrow. The angle of the femoral neck (*anteversion*) may be abnormally high. Custom components may be needed in these situations. Additional reconstruction, such as shortening of the femur to bring the hip back to its natural socket, may be necessary.

In Perthes disease, the femoral head may be wide and flat, and the neck of the femur may be unusually large. The acetabulum may be deformed to accommodate the abnormal shape of the femoral head. All of these changes need to be considered when the surgeon plans his procedure.

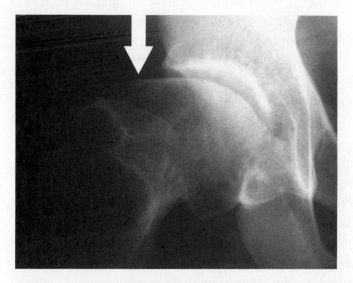

Figure 7   X-ray of hip with arthritis secondary to SCFE. The neck of the femur (arrow) has a round prominent shape.

In SCFE the femoral neck may be deformed and sometimes rotated backward (retroverted). Patients with this disease may turn their leg outward or have an external rotation gait. They have frequently undergone a surgical procedure such as pinning or osteotomy as part of treatment for the disease. Both the deformity and the hardware are factors when surgery is planned.

While the symptoms of these diseases are similar to those of osteoarthritis, hip replacement can be more challenging due to the variable anatomy.

11. What other conditions can cause arthritis in my hip?

Several other conditions can damage the hip joint and lead to hip replacement.

A previous infection in the hip joint may cause long-term changes that lead to arthritis. An infected joint during childhood or a bone infection, *osteomyelitis*, can injure the growing bony surfaces. A patient who has had an infection as a child or teenager may develop arthritis when he or she becomes an adult.

Infection after previous hip surgery can also cause arthritis. The infection can erode cartilage and destroy the joint.

A low-grade infection can persist for a long period of time, even years, in bone. When an infection develops after surgery, bacteria may remain in bone even though the infection appears to be treated.

If hip replacement is planned on a hip that was once infected, testing should be done to make sure no active infection remains.

Hemophilia is a disease where absence of a clotting factor (mostly factor VIII or XI) causes abnormal bleeding. Patients with hemophilia have bleeding into a joint or **hemarthrosis**. This causes a process that results in destruction of the joint.

The hip is less affected by hemophilia than the knees or ankles, but disease can still occur. When hip replacement surgery is performed, the missing clotting factor must be replaced before surgery. An appropriate level of clotting factor should be maintained during surgery and in the postoperative period.

Ankylosing spondylitis is a condition that develops in young men between teenage years and age 40 years. It causes fusion of joints, particularly in the pelvis and spine. Joints in the rib cage that allow the chest wall to expand when breathing are also involved. A special blood test, HLA-B27, can help make the diagnosis when it is positive. A hip joint with ankylosing spondylitis can develop arthritis with symptoms that are similar to osteoarthritis. The hip usually fuses in a bent or flexed position.

Gaucher's disease is a storage disease. Due to a metabolic disorder, abnormal amounts of fatty material are deposited or stored in different organs of the body. These include liver, spleen, brain and bone marrow. The fatty deposits in the bone marrow can cause avascular necrosis of the femoral head and eventually arthritis. Like hemophilia, Gaucher's disease is a genetic disorder that can be passed on from one generation to the next.

Sickle cell anemia is found predominantly in African Americans or people of African descent. Under certain

Hemophilia

A disease where absence of a clotting factor in the blood causes abnormal bleeding.

Hemarthrosis

Bleeding into a joint that often occurs with hemophilia.

Ankylosing spondylitis

Condition that develops in young men between teenage years and age 40, which causes fusion of joints, particularly in the pelvis and spine.

Gaucher's disease

A metabolic disease that can cause avascular necrosis. Abnormal amounts of fatty material are deposited in different organs of the body.

Sickle cell anemia

A disease found predominantly in African Americans or people of African descent. Round red blood cells take on a crescent or sickle shape and cannot pass through small vessels in the body. This can cause avascular necrosis in the hip.

conditions, the normally round red blood cells take on a crescent or sickle shape and cannot pass through small vessels in the body. Blood supply to tissues is blocked. Patients can experience painful sickle cell crises.

In bone, sickle cell disease causes areas of bone death or *infarcts*. This leads to avascular necrosis in the femoral head. When hip replacement is performed, measures must be taken to prevent a sickle cell crisis during the procedure.

Paget's disease

A metabolic disease of bone where bone is rapidly destroyed and then repaired. The rapid rate of bone metabolism causes abnormal appearance and bone deformity.

Paget's disease is a metabolic disease of bone. Bone is rapidly destroyed and then repaired. It can involve one or several bones at a time. It most often affects the spine, pelvis, and long bones, such as the humerus or femur. The rapid rate of bone metabolism causes deformity and abnormal appearance of the bone. Sometimes stress fractures may develop.

Paget's disease can cause osteoarthritis of the hip. The abnormal anatomy and bone structure may make hip replacement more difficult.

PART THREE

Symptoms

Why does my hip hurt? Where does it hurt?

Why do I limp? Why does my leg feel short?

Why does my hip sometimes make a crackling noise
when I try to move it?

More . . .

12. Why does my hip hurt? Where does it hurt?

An arthritic hip is painful because the joint has broken down. The articular cartilage on the surfaces of the joint has worn away leaving raw bone exposed. Movement between the two joint surfaces is no longer smooth and friction free. As a result, the tissues within the joint become inflamed and the joint begins to hurt. An excess amount of joint fluid may be produced and the resultant swelling of the joint adds to the symptoms.

The exposed raw bony surfaces have a greater nerve supply than the articular cartilage and pressure on these surfaces causes pain. As the joint becomes stiffer, greater strain is placed on the hip muscles as they move the joint. This too can be painful. The friction between the exposed bony surfaces can cause grinding and a feeling of discomfort.

When the joint is inflamed, there may be pain both with activity and when the joint is at rest.

When the joint is inflamed, there may be pain both with activity and when the joint is at rest. Anatomically, the hip joint fits deep in the groin. For this reason, groin pain may be the first sign of an arthritic hip. The pain may radiate to the outside or lateral side of the hip or to the back or posterior aspect of the hip. It will often extend to the mid portion of the thigh and down to the knee. Since the ball of the hip, the femoral head, is part of the femur the pain travels down the length of the entire bone and will be felt in the thigh and the knee.

When the pain goes below the knee, it is often a sign of a different problem, such as sciatica or poor circulation.

13. When will I have pain?

An arthritic hip can hurt at any time. Much of the time pain will occur after prolonged standing, walking, or any other weight bearing activity. It may also come from activities that put stress on the hip such as bending, twisting, running, and climbing stairs.

Sometimes the pain may develop spontaneously and be present when you are doing nothing at all. This is called resting pain. Frequently, this kind of pain can occur at night and can awaken you from sleep.

People who have osteoarthritis will sometimes complain of pain in an affected joint when there is a change in the weather. An episode of pain may last for several days and then recede. It is not clear what triggers the inflammatory response that causes the pain.

In many people with advanced osteoarthritis, the pain is constant and is present all the time. It is unrelieved by rest, by any change in position, or by medication.

Linda W., a patient, says:

The pain was a constant burning pain. Nothing relieved the pain—not rest, ibuprofen, or even more potent medications. The medications would sort of deaden the pain, allowing me to get to sleep, but I would wake up during the night and have to change positions.

The time to consider hip replacement surgery is when you can no longer tolerate the pain.

14. Why do I limp? Why does my leg feel short?

Limping means an abnormal gait or walking pattern. Limping may come from a variety of causes such as pain, deformity or shortening of the leg. It can also come from a neurologic cause such as paralysis of some of the muscles in the leg.

The time to consider hip replacement surgery is when you can no longer tolerate the pain.

Antalgic

A limping gait that avoids pain.

The major cause of limping in an arthritic hip is pain. A gait that avoids pain is said to be **antalgic**. This happens because you attempt to put less weight on the painful hip. You try to spend less time bearing weight on that side. You may also take shorter steps as you try to minimize the time you put on your bad leg.

As you lose movement, your hip becomes stiffer. Your leg may turn inward (internally rotated) or outward (externally rotated) and develop a fixed rotational deformity. Shortening may result from either a flexion contracture of the hip or loss of height as the joint surfaces collapse. Your leg may also feel short if you have spinal problems and your pelvis is tilted. Thus, an abnormal gait may have more than one component in an arthritic hip. For example, your gait may be described as short leg, flexed hip, antalgic, and rotated.

A neurologic problem such as peripheral neuropathy or polio can cause weakness of the muscles of the leg and an abnormal gait. A neurologic problem may not be directly connected to an arthritic hip, but the resultant gait problem has to be considered if you are planning total hip arthroplasty.

Patients with a bad hip will often have a *Trendelenburg gait*. This means the body tilts sideways over the bad hip as they attempt to go forward. Using a cane may improve or eliminate this portion of an abnormal gait.

15. Why can't I bend over? Why can't I tie my shoes?

When your hip is arthritic, it may become stiff. Since the motion in your hip is restricted, you will have difficulty doing some of the things you did before.

Even when you don't have pain, the symptoms of stiffness may be limiting.

At first, you may have trouble bending over to pick up objects. You may have to stoop down and bend your knees in order to reach the floor. You may notice difficulty getting in and out of your car or you may have difficulty getting up from a low chair. It may be hard to bend over to cut your toenails, to put on your socks or to tie your shoes. At first, you may find yourself bending your leg in an awkward position in order to accomplish these things. Then you may be unable to do them at all. Additional aids such as a grabber or shoehorn might be helpful. As time passes, you may even have difficulty getting dressed.

When your hip has lost motion it is harder to do stairs in an alternating pattern. You may need to go up with your good leg first and down with your bad leg. It may take longer to put your leg down on the floor when you first get out of a chair.

All of these are signs of stiffness of the hip. This occurs because the muscles and ligaments around the hip contract as arthritis becomes more advanced. When the muscles and joint capsule tighten, you lose range of motion. The hip goes into a flexed position and develops a *flexion contracture*. You will no longer be able to move your hip the way you once did. Your range of activities may become restricted.

If your hip is stiff you may compensate by putting pressure on your spine. This can cause lower back pain. You may also have increased pain in your knee if your knee is arthritic.

Even when you don't have pain, the symptoms of stiffness may be limiting.

Symptoms

16. Why does my hip sometimes make a crackling noise when I try to move it?

A crackling or snapping of the hip joint can be disconcerting. It feels uncomfortable and it makes a loud noise that sometimes other people in the room can hear. The medical term for crackling or snapping is *crepitus*.

In simplest terms, crepitus occurs because bone is rubbing against bone. The joint cartilage has broken down and the joint surfaces become irregular. When this happens, the joint no longer moves smoothly. There is friction between the two bones. The joint may catch or get stuck momentarily before it starts to move again. Crepitus is often painful when the hip joint gets stuck. It may make you stop in your tracks as you are trying to move forward. It may make it especially hard for you to go up and down stairs.

Factors other than osteoarthritis can cause crepitus. Sometimes, the presence of a loose body or fragment of bone or cartilage moving in the joint can cause momentary friction. You can also get a grinding sensation if there is disruption in the joint surface such as from an old fracture.

The presence of crepitus in an arthritic joint is usually a sign that arthritis is advanced and will soon require hip replacement.

PART FOUR

Diagnosis

How will my doctor make the diagnosis
of an arthritic hip?

Do I need an MRI?

What is an arthrogram? When is it done?

More . . .

17. How will my doctor make the diagnosis of an arthritic hip?

When you go to your orthopaedic surgeon, he will take several steps to make the diagnosis. While the presence of an arthritic hip may seem obvious to you, your surgeon will need to evaluate your hip to make sure the diagnosis is correct.

First, he will take a history of your problem. He or she will want to know where you have pain, how long it has been present and when it started. He will want to know if the pain developed on its own or came after an injury. He may ask you what part of your hip or your leg hurts and what movements make it hurt.

Tell your surgeon if you are limping or you are having trouble walking. He will ask if you have difficulty with certain activities such as bending over, tying your shoes or going up and down stairs. Tell him how much pain medicine you take and whether anything makes the pain better or worse.

Part of your history includes any hip problems or injury in the past. Your surgeon will want to know if you have had childhood hip disease, a fracture, or some other condition that might cause pain in your hip. He will also want to hear about any condition that causes arthritis throughout your body.

You should also discuss your family history. If, for example, both your mother and grandmother had arthritis in their hips, then you might be suffering from a similar problem.

When your surgeon completes the history, he will do a physical examination. This involves checking for tenderness or deformity around your hip. He will test the range of motion of your hip joint, evaluate the strength in your leg, and watch how you stand and walk. He may also look at other areas such as your spine which could cause pain in your hip.

In addition to history and physical examination, an x-ray will help make the diagnosis. If the disease is far enough advanced, an x-ray will show the changes of an arthritic hip. It may also provide a clue as to what has caused the arthritis such as an old fracture or a childhood hip problem. An x-ray along with your history and physical findings will most often confirm the diagnosis.

Sometimes, the plain x-ray may not show the problem. When this happens, the surgeon may choose to obtain *a Magnetic Resonance Imaging* study, or *MRI*. MRI can show a stress fracture or avascular necrosis when the early changes are not always evident on a plain film.

Your surgeon may order a blood test to rule out a systemic problem such as rheumatoid arthritis. Other blood tests might help diagnose problems such as infection, lupus, or ankylosing spondylitis.

Finally, he may ask that you have an **aspiration** done to retrieve fluid from your hip. This is done by a radiologist under x-ray guidance. A sample of the hip joint fluid would be taken and sent to the laboratory for evaluation and for culture to make sure that there is no infection.

Aspiration
A procedure done by needle puncture to remove fluid from a joint.

Once your doctor has made the diagnosis of an arthritic hip, he will present you with the range of treatment options.

18. What will my doctor find when he does an examination?

Physical examination is very helpful to your doctor in making the diagnosis of a painful hip.

He or she will examine how you stand, how you walk, and how you move. He will check the alignment of your spine and pelvis and look to make sure they are level.

If your pelvis is tilted, it might be a sign that your hip pain is due to a back problem. Limited motion of your spine may also suggest that your back is the real cause of your pain.

Your doctor may then ask you to lie down flat on your back on an examining table. He will first examine your legs to make sure that they appear equal. He may check the circular measurement of the thigh, the circumference, against the opposite side. If one leg is smaller or thinner than the other, it may be a sign of *atrophy* of the muscle, which causes thinning and weakness. This may be due to chronic hip disease. It may also be a sign of a chronic neurologic problem that has caused wasting or thinning of the muscle.

Your surgeon may also want to measure the length of both of your legs. This can be done in two ways. The first of these, **apparent leg length** measures the length of your leg but can be affected by the angle of your pelvis. A measurement is taken with a tape measure from your umbilicus to the *medial malleolus* on the inner part of your ankle. The second measurement is called **true leg length**. This measures the length of your leg without regard to any pelvic tilting or deformity. This is measured from a bony prominence on the

Your surgeon may also want to measure the length of both of your legs.

Apparent leg length

A measurement of leg length taken from the umbilicus to the medial malleolus that can be affected by tilting or contraction of the pelvis.

True leg length

A measurement of the length of leg without regard to tilting or deformity of the pelvis. The measurement is taken from a point on the front of the pelvis called the anterior superior iliac spine to the medial malleolus.

front of your pelvis called the *anterior superior iliac spine* to the same point as before, the medial malleolus, on the inner side of your ankle.

Your surgeon will compare the leg lengths he measures from the right side to the left side. If there is a difference it may be due to the fact that the hip is shortened from ongoing arthritis or disease. It may also be important when your surgeon performs your hip replacement. By knowing the difference between the two or the *leg length discrepancy,* he may be able to restore your leg to its normal length. This will be very important as you walk.

Leg length discrepancy may also be caused by other factors such as previous injury to the leg, an old fracture, or shortening at birth known as *congenital* shortening.

If, however, there are no other reasons for a leg length discrepancy, then shortening may be a sign of an arthritic hip. The shortening due to arthritis is usually in the range of 1 to 2 cm for an adult.

Your doctor will next want to check to see if there is a hip flexion contracture. This means that the hip has become stiff due to arthritis and cannot fully straighten. If you have a flexion contracture, any attempts to straighten your hip and leg may cause pain or may cause your spine to move.

Your surgeon will perform the *Thomas test*. He will flatten your spine on the table by flexing your opposite hip. He will then attempt to straighten or *extend* your bad hip. If your leg cannot come fully flat on the table, it means that it is permanently flexed or has a flexion contracture.

A flexion contracture can make your leg seem shorter when you stand and walk. This is part of an apparent leg length discrepancy.

Your doctor will next measure range of motion in other directions or planes. Limited range of motion may be a sign of an arthritic or diseased hip. He will first *flex* your hip. That is, he will attempt to bend your leg up towards the rest of your body. The point at which your hip stops bending is the range of *flexion*. Typically, a hip with arthritis will have limitation of both flexion and extension.

Your doctor will then check the range of *rotation*. Rotation can be tested in two directions, internal and external. Internal rotation is when the thigh is turned inward so that the foot points away from the body. External rotation is the reverse. Patients with an arthritic hip often have limitation of internal rotation. It may be both limited and painful.

Your surgeon will also test the range of *adduction* and *abduction*. Adduction is bringing your leg over the midline of your body as if it would cross the other leg. Abduction means bring your leg away from your body as if you were doing a split. A diseased hip may show limitation of motion in both directions. Adduction is often painful.

Your surgeon will look for swelling in other joints. This might be a sign of another disease process such as rheumatoid arthritis or Lyme disease. He will check the range of motion in your knees and ankles and look for any deformities in your feet. If movement of these joints causes pain in your leg, your surgeon may want to take x-rays or do further investigation.

A peripheral neurologic examination of your leg is important. This is done to make sure that there are no associated neurologic conditions causing pain. Your doctor will do a straight leg raise test and check the sensation and motor strength of your leg. He may also test the reflexes.

He will feel the pulses in your legs and feet. This is to make sure that your have adequate circulation. Poor circulation can cause pain in your thigh and leg and may limit your walking. If there are no pulses, arterial disease should be ruled out as a cause of pain. It is critical to make sure that blood circulation in the leg is adequate if surgery is being planned.

Your doctor may perform a *Trendelenburg* test. He will ask you first to stand and balance on your good leg and then to do the same on the bad leg. If you are unable to balance on your bad leg, your body will tip to the side. This is a positive test. It indicates weak muscles around your hip, a sign of hip disease.

Your doctor will examine the way you walk and perform an evaluation of your gait. If you have a flexion contracture, you may walk with a flexed hip and you may lean forward on your bad hip as you walk. You may also demonstrate an abductor lurch where your body tips to the side of your bad hip. Most patients with painful hips will show a limping or antalgic gait. If disease is severe, you may require a cane or other assistive aids to walk at all.

Physical findings may depend somewhat on the type of disease and degree of involvement in the hip. For example, patients with advanced osteoarthritis will have a flexion contracture and severely limited range of

A peripheral neurologic examination of your leg is important. This is done to make sure that there are no associated neurologic conditions causing pain.

Diagnosis

motion. There may even be audible noise, or crepitus, as the hip is moved.

On the other hand, patients with avascular necrosis may have severe pain with movement but relatively good range of motion until the final stages of the disease.

Patients who have been treated for dislocated hips in childhood may have shortening and a leg that is internally rotated. Others who have been treated for slipped capital femoral epiphysis during the teenage years may have an external rotation gait and turn their legs outward as they walk.

If a patient has had polio or other neurologic disease for many years, the leg may be shortened and the muscles weak. This may affect all joints of the leg not only the hip.

Your doctor's physical examination can provide many clues as to the nature of the problem in your hip and help him make a better diagnosis.

19. What do x-rays show?

Your doctor will want to see x-rays of your hip as part of your office consultation. If you bring x-rays with you, he will want to review them. If not, he may take x-rays in his office. If your x-rays are several months old, he may want to take new pictures because your hip may have changed. X-rays of a hip with arthritis will be different from a normal hip. They may be used to confirm the diagnosis.

Typically, two x-rays are taken of the hip joint in different positions. An *AP* view shows the front of the hip. A *lateral* view shows the hip from the side.

If you have symptoms in your opposite hip as well your doctor may want to obtain x-rays of the pelvis or of both hips.

In a normal x-ray, the ball of the femur, the femoral head, is smooth and round. The neck of the femur is the long section below the ball. The bone inside the femoral head and femoral neck has a uniform cross-hatched or **trabecular** pattern. A notch on the surface of the ball, the *fovea*, is where blood vessels enter the femoral head.

The hip joint socket or acetabulum is opposite the femoral head. Like the surface of the femoral head the socket is round. It covers almost, but not all, of the ball of the femur on an AP or frontal view. In a normal hip the ball is well-centered in the socket.

The space between the ball and socket appears to be clear. This is because the surfaces of the joint are covered by **hyaline cartilage**. Unlike bone, normal cartilage does not have any calcium. Therefore, it cannot be seen on x-ray and looks like a clear empty space.

In a hip with arthritis, the cartilage is worn down and the space between the two joint surfaces is smaller or narrowed. When the arthritis is severe the clear space is completely gone and the two joint surfaces appear to be rubbing against each other. The joint is said to be *bone on bone*. Sometimes it looks as if the ball and socket are fused together.

The head of the femur may become deformed and the surface may have a flattened appearance.

In long standing cases, the bone may become hard or *sclerotic*. It will have a dense whitish look on x-ray.

In a normal x-ray, the ball of the femur, the femoral head, is smooth and round.

Trabecular
A cross-hatched pattern seen on an x-ray in the bone of the femoral head and femoral neck.

Hyaline cartilage
The type of cartilage that covers joint surfaces.

Bony projections form at the edges of the femoral head. These are called bone spurs or *osteophytes*.

In rare cases, x-rays may show that the ball has pushed completely through the socket and into the pelvis. This is called *protrusio*.

X-rays may help to distinguish arthritis from avascular necrosis. They can also reveal unusual conditions in the hip such as *Paget's disease* or bone tumors. In Paget's disease the bone becomes dense and deformed. The trabecular lines of the bone become whitish and sclerotic.

Pathologic fracture

A fracture which occurs through abnormal bone such as a bone cyst, Paget's disease, or cancer.

Bone tumors may appear as a clear area (*lytic*) or as an area of dense growing bone (*blastic*). A tumor may even cause a **pathologic fracture** of the bone.

Template

A tracing or outline of different sized hip components placed over an x-ray before surgery to estimate the size and position of the implants in a hip replacement.

Your orthopaedic surgeon will use the x-rays to confirm the diagnosis and determine the severity of the disease. He may also use the x-rays as a **template**. He will take measurements that determine what size components will be used and where in the bone they will be placed. While a template may not be exact, it provides a guide or road map for the surgeon to use during surgery.

20. Do I need an MRI?

Most often the diagnosis of osteoarthritis of the hip can be made on a plain x-ray. Joint space narrowing, deformity, and spur formation are much more obvious on a plain film than on an MRI.

MRI is used to diagnose certain problems in the hip which may cause pain similar to osteoarthritis.

MRI is used to diagnose certain problems in the hip which may cause pain similar to osteoarthritis.

MRI stands for Magnetic Resonance Imaging. When the technology was first developed, it was known as

Nuclear Magnetic Resonance. The name was changed, however, because it was felt that the word *nuclear* implied the use of radioactive material. In fact, there is no radioactivity with an MRI scanner at all.

MRI has been utilized in orthopaedic surgery for more than 20 years. It is done mostly to evaluate soft tissue problems and ligament injuries but can be helpful in diagnosing problems of bones and joints as well.

In the hip, several problems are often diagnosed first by MRI.

1. Avascular necrosis

   In its early stages, avascular necrosis is often not seen on a plain x-ray. The earliest changes of AVN in the femoral head are subtle changes in the bone which are best seen on an MRI. If AVN is diagnosed early enough and the femoral head has not collapsed, a *core decompression* procedure may be done and the hip joint preserved.

2. Fractures

   A fracture of the hip may be visible as fluid or edema within the bone before it can be seen as a fracture line on plain x-ray. In some situations, spontaneous stress fractures of the neck of the femur can cause pain in the groin and thigh similar to osteoarthritis. Stress fractures may be seen in young, active patients who are runners or in older patients with thin or osteoporotic bone. The pain of a spontaneous fracture may be similar to the pain of an arthritic hip and an MRI may be very useful in making the diagnosis.

3. Transient osteoporosis

   Transient osteoporosis of the hip is an inflammation of the head and neck of the femur that can cause acute pain similar to that of osteoarthritis. Transient osteoporosis develops spontaneously and resolves in several months. MRI will show fluid or edema in a wide area of the bone. A plain x-ray, however, will be normal. This condition almost always resolves spontaneously with no need for surgery.

4. Tumors

Bone tumors may be detected on MRI before they are seen on plain x-ray. A bone tumor may show subtle changes in the marrow of the bone which are best visualized on MRI. A tumor may be diagnosed and treatment begun in an early stage.

5. **Septic arthritis**

Septic arthritis
Infection in a joint.

If there is a large amount of fluid or pus in the joint, it is best seen on an MRI. This may help make the diagnosis of infection in the joint or *septic arthritis*.

MRI may thus be helpful in diagnosing conditions not well seen on a plain x-ray. Most often, the diagnosis of osteoarthritis is clear, but sometimes an MRI can be helpful.

Some patients cannot have an MRI because of medical implants or metallic fragments within their bodies.

Some patients cannot have an MRI because of medical implants or metallic fragments within their bodies. Patients who have a pacemaker or defibrillator, a cochlear implant in the ear, or surgical clips following surgery for a brain aneurysm cannot have an MRI. MRI can also not be done if there are small metal fragments within your body near vital organs such as the eyes.

Most orthopaedic implants such as joint replacements, plates, and screws are not affected by an MRI and do not prevent a patient from having the study.

Diagnosis

21. What is an arthrogram? When is it done?

An arthrogram is a procedure where radiopaque dye or contrast is injected into the joint and plain x-rays are taken. It is done to diagnose infection or **loosening**.

Joint fluid can be removed and sent to the laboratory for culture. In this way, it can be determined if there are any bacteria or there is an infection in the joint.

If there is loosening of one of the components, the contrast material will penetrate the space around the component between the component and the bone. This is a sign that the component is loose and has separated from bone.

In some circumstances, an MRI may be combined with a contrast injection procedure. This is called an *MR arthrogram*.

22. Can I have pain in my hip from other problems?

When the diagnosis of an arthritic hip is not clear, it is important to consider other problems that might cause similar pain in the groin and thigh.

Problems in the lumbar spine, such as disc herniation and spinal stenosis, can cause pain in the hip. This is because the nerve roots that supply feeling to the hip are affected by the disease.

A disc herniation or **herniated nucleus pulposus** can cause hip pain if it presses a nerve root on the affected side. By the same token, spinal stenosis which also causes inflammation of the nerve roots, can mimic the symptoms of an arthritic hip. It is important to consider

Loosening

When one or both components of a hip replacement is no longer securely fixed to bone.

Herniated nucleus pulposus (Herniated Disc)

A condition where disc material between vertebrae extrudes into the spinal canal causing pressure on nerve roots and leg pain.

both of these diagnoses, especially in patients who have a history of spinal problems.

Clinically, there are several ways to separate spinal disease from hip disease. In a disc herniation, the pain will be radicular; that is, it will extend down the leg. There may be some loss of feeling or weakness of the muscles and loss of a reflex. Straight leg raise test will often be positive. There will, however, be normal range of motion of the hip, and movement of the joint itself will not be painful. In an arthritic hip, joint motion will be both limited and painful.

MRI of the spine will show the disc herniation and confirm the diagnosis.

Spinal stenosis usually develops after age 50 years. As with disc herniation, pressure on the L2 or L3 nerve roots can cause pain in the hip. Stenosis pain, however, usually develops after an individual has been walking for several minutes. It begins as a burning or numbing and then becomes pain. It is completely relieved when the individual sits down to rest. Physical examination in spinal stenosis is often unremarkable. Again, this contrasts to an arthritic hip where motion is limited and painful. As with other spinal problems, MRI can be used to confirm the diagnosis.

Some situations require a frank discussion between doctor and patient as to which problem is more symptomatic and which should be treated first.

Some elderly patients have symptoms and radiographic findings of both an arthritic hip and spinal stenosis. When this occurs, it is important to determine the primary cause of pain. Some situations require a frank discussion between doctor and patient as to which problem is more symptomatic and which should be treated first. It is important to realize that no matter which problem is treated, some symptoms will remain.

Neuropathy, like disc herniation and spinal stenosis, is a neurological problem. In neuropathy, however, the nerve itself is inflamed rather than being compressed. It is sometimes present in patients with diabetes mellitus. Neuropathy can cause hip or thigh pain, but examination of the hip will again be normal. If neuropathy is suspected, consultation with a neurologist will be obtained.

Arterial insufficiency or narrowing of one of the main arteries in the leg can cause pain in the hip and thigh. Most often, symptoms are in the lower leg, but they can occur closer to the hip. Arterial problems can be easily diagnosed by the absence of pulses or by tests that measure the blood flow to the leg.

Other causes of hip pain include inguinal hernia, urologic problems, and gynecologic disease. Pain localized to the groin can sometimes be caused by an inguinal hernia. This can be easily detected on physical examination by either your family physician or a general surgeon. Urologic problems such as prostate disease may also cause pain that radiates to the groin area. In this case, evaluation and testing by an urologist can help to diagnose the problem.

Finally, some pelvic problems such endometriosis can cause pain in the area of the hip and can be diagnosed by a gynecologist.

PART FIVE

Treatment Without Surgery

Will it help to lose weight?

What are NSAIDs?

Do supplements like Glucosamine help?

More . . .

23. Should I limit my activity? Can exercise help?

If you have arthritis, it is important to keep your hip joint mobile. Over time, the arthritis will progress. Your hip will feel stiffer and you will lose range of motion. It is therefore helpful to try to do everything you can to maintain the range of motion in your hip. You will walk better and be able to enjoy more of your regular activities and sports. A good exercise program will help preserve both the strength and the motion in your hip. Strengthening the muscles around your hip and thigh can take some of the pressure off your arthritic joint.

A good exercise program will help preserve both the strength and the motion in your hip.

If you are planning surgery, strengthening the muscles around your hip will make your recovery easier.

Staying active is an important part of living with an arthritic hip. There is no evidence that limiting your activity will stop the progression of arthritis. Let your pain and level of comfort be your guide as to what you can and cannot do.

If you have any questions, a physical therapist can help you set up a regular exercise program for your hip.

24. Will it help to lose weight?

Most individuals planning hip replacement surgery do not need to worry about weight.

If you are very overweight, then losing weight before surgery may be helpful. Under the best of circumstances, it is hard to trim even a few pounds. If your hip is painful, it is even more difficult to move about and to exercise. This makes weight loss all the more difficult. Nevertheless, being overweight does present certain problems for surgery.

An overweight patient with a large amount of soft tissue around the hip requires a longer incision and wider surgical exposure to reach the hip joint. This means increased surgical time and often a greater blood loss. More retraction is required during surgery and this puts deeper structures such as the sciatic nerve at risk.

Overweight patients have a greater tendency towards wound healing problems which may lead to infection.

In the postoperative period, extra weight makes physical therapy and mobility more difficult. Heavier patients are at higher risk for medical complications such as blood clots and thrombophlebitis. Since they have greater difficulty breathing and moving air, there may be an increased incidence of lung problems. Overweight patients as a group may also have a greater risk of diabetes.

In short, overweight patients are more likely to have medical problems in the postoperative period. The good news is that there is no proven difference in recovery time and no known difference in orthopaedic surgical outcomes between normal and overweight patients. Surprisingly, there is nothing to suggest a higher risk of instability in overweight patients. They may, in fact, be protected because they are unable to flex their hips as much. We can therefore say that being overweight carries a greater risk of postoperative medical problems, but the overall orthopaedic results are the same. If your weight is a concern, your regular physician and your orthopaedic surgeon can tell you what steps need to be taken before you have surgery.

25. Should I use a cane?

When you have a bad hip you may find it helpful to use a cane. A cane can help take some of the weight off of your hip, it can help you balance and may enable you to walk greater distances.

The cane lets you put some of the weight on your good side, which would otherwise fall on your bad hip and cause you to limp. Without the cane, your body may be unable to balance and may list to one side as you step forward. Mechanically, it is best to use the cane in the hand opposite the side of your bad hip. Try it on both sides, but you will find that the opposite side works best. Using the cane on the opposite side allows you to transfer weight to the good side and to walk more easily.

It is best to use the cane in the hand opposite the side of your bad hip.

If your hip pain is not too bad, you may only want to use the cane for walking long distances. As the disease becomes more advanced, you may want to use the cane all the time.

Most people use a cane with a single tip, a *straight cane*. A *quad cane* has a platform at the base and four tips called prongs. This may have greater stability if your balance is poor. Many people choose to use a four prong cane during the time when they are recovering from surgery.

If the pain becomes really severe, then you may even consider using crutches or a walker.

Remember that a cane can help you walk and go about your daily activities, but it does not truly relieve the arthritis pain.

26. What are NSAIDs?

NSAID's are nonsteroidal anti-inflammatory drugs. They are the most common treatment for arthritis and painful joints. NSAIDs can be taken orally.

Unlike steroids, NSAIDs do not occur naturally in the human body. They are chemically synthesized medications, which have a similar anti-inflammatory effect. They also do not produce the side effects associated with prolonged steroid therapy.

NSAIDs relieve pain, reduce fever, and prevent inflammation. They work by inhibiting the action of the enzyme *cyclooxygenase*, which helps produce *prostaglandins* throughout the body. Prostaglandins stimulate the inflammatory response in an arthritic joint. By limiting the action of cyclooxygenase, NSAIDs can reduce inflammation.

There are two cyclooxygenase enzymes, *COX-1* and *COX-2*. COX-2 is the mediator of the inflammatory response. COX-1 protects the lining of the stomach. An NSAID that affects both of these enzymes will reduce inflammation but also cause gastric or stomach upset. Most NSAIDs block the action of COX-1 and COX-2. Some drugs are more selective and are COX-2 inhibitors only.

Aspirin is the oldest and most common NSAID. Its chemical name is acetylsalicylic acid and was first synthesized more than 100 years ago. It is now available as a generic product from several companies. Aspirin also helps to prevent the action of platelets in the blood. It is the only NSAID that inhibits clotting. Some aspirin preparations are buffered to protect the stomach.

NSAIDs can be effective in relieving the pain of an arthritic joint. Their most common side effect is gastric upset. There are also risks of kidney damage, allergic response, and interference with blood pressure medication. Among the NSAIDs, aspirin is also known to cause tinnitus or ringing in the ears.

NSAIDs can be taken on a regular or on an intermittent basis. If you find an NSAID that works for you, you may only want to take the medication on a bad day. This might be a day when you are planning to walk long distances, to participate in sports or to be dancing at a party or family event. As your arthritis gets worse, however, you may need to take the medication on a regular basis.

Not all NSAIDs work for every patient. You may, in fact, need to try several different drugs before you find one that is effective for you.

You should not take NSAIDs if you have a history of stomach or intestinal problems, a blood clotting disorder, you are on blood thinners, you are pregnant, or you are breast feeding. Make sure your doctor is aware of any medical conditions you might have before you start taking NSAIDs.

If you cannot take NSAIDs, acetaminophen (Tylenol) may be an option. Tylenol is not considered an NSAID because it does not have an anti-inflammatory effect. It does, however, relieve pain and bring down fever. Its main side effect is liver damage when it is taken for a long period of time. Tylenol should not be taken if you are already taking an NSAID medication.

Some of the more common NSAIDs are:

- Aspirin
- Enteric-coated aspirin (Ecotrin)
- Celecoxib (Celebrex)
- Diclofenac (Voltaren)
- Diflunisal (Dolobid)
- Etodolac (Lodine)
- Ibuprofen (Motrin, Advil)
- Indomethacin (Indocin)
- Ketoprofen (Orudis)
- Ketorolac (Toradol)
- Nabumetone (Relafen)
- Naproxen (Aleve, Naprosyn)
- Oxaprozin (Daypro)
- Piroxicam (Feldene)
- Sulindac (Clinoril)
- Tolmctin (Tolectin)
- Meloxicam (Mobic)

All of these drugs have similar action and similar side effects. They can be helpful in treating the symptoms of an arthritic hip if you are not yet ready for surgery.

27. Do supplements like Glucosamine help?

Glucosamine and Chondroitin are substances that occur naturally within the human body. They help to build and maintain the structure of normal articular cartilage in a joint. For this reason, many people take Glucosamine and Chondroitin in the hope that they will prevent arthritis from progressing or getting any worse.

Glucosamine is a substance made from glucose (sugar) and an amino acid called glutamine. It is used to form glycosaminoglycan. This is a substance that helps build cartilage in the human body.

Chondroitin is found in articular cartilage. It protects the cartilage from breakdown by enzymes within the joint.

Some people feel that taken together Glucosamine and Chondroitin can prevent destruction of the joint and delay the symptoms of arthritis.

Glucosamine and Chondroitin are classified as dietary or nutritional supplements. They are not medications. They are sold over the counter and are not regulated by the Food & Drug Administration. Many companies produce and sell different combinations of Glucosamine and Chondroitin. The dosage and ingredients in each preparation cannot be verified. Often the ingredients of Glucosamine may be extracted from shellfish such as crab or lobster. Patients with known shellfish allergies should be careful about taking Glucosamine. It may be helpful to get information from the manufacturer.

The most common daily dose of Glucosamine is 1500 mg per day split into two or three divided doses. Chondroitin is taken in a daily dose of 1200 mg per day, again divided into two or three doses. These may be reduced over time if the combination seems to be effective.

High doses of these supplements may cause side effects. These include headache, drowsiness, and gastrointestinal symptoms such as nausea, diarrhea, or stomach upset. Patients who have diabetes mellitus should also have their glucose levels carefully monitored.

Thus far, most of the evidence for or against the use of Glucosamine and Chondroitin is anecdotal.

Thus far, most of the evidence for or against the use of Glucosamine and Chondroitin is anecdotal. They may have an anti-inflammatory affect and thus give relief of pain. There are, however, no large scientific studies that show any permanent effects on the articular cartilage.

There is no evidence that they slow the progress of arthritis or actually repair the cartilage.

The long-term effects of taking Glucosamine and Chondroitin are not known. They should be taken as a supplement but not as a substitute for your regular arthritis treatment. If you have any questions about taking these supplements, it is best to talk to your doctor.

28. Can a cortisone injection help?

Cortisone or corticosteroid injections can sometimes provide short-term relief for inflammatory symptoms in many joints of the body. Cortisone is a naturally occurring substance within the body. Injectable steroid preparations can sometimes relieve the pain of an arthritic hip.

Cortisone injections can be easily given to large joints such as the knee and shoulder and smaller joints such as the ankle and elbow because parts of the joint are right beneath the skin. All of these joints have a surface which can be easily felt and penetrated with a needle. The hip joint however is very deep within the body. In order to reach the hip joint, a needle must go through several layers of muscle and the joint capsule.

The hip joint is largely covered by the round dome of the socket or acetabulum. Only a small portion of the joint can be penetrated with a needle. Since it is deep, this cannot be done easily.

Hip injections are therefore most often done by a radiologist. Use of a continuous x-ray or fluoroscopy is helpful in making sure that the needle and the medication enter the joint. Once the position of the needle has been confirmed, the medication can be safely injected.

Usually, this is a small dose of a steroid preparation which stays within the joint. Steroids can provide good short-term relief, which may last anywhere from a few days to several months. If the injection relieves the pain even only in the short term, it is a good sign that the arthritic joint is the cause of the symptoms.

Steroid injections are not done very often in the hip and too many injections can ultimately cause long-term damage.

PART SIX

Surgery

Can I have a total hip replacement if I have had previous hip surgery?

What is Bipolar (Partial) Hip Replacement?

What is resurfacing?

More . . .

29. Can I be too young to have hip replacement surgery?

For many years, surgeons felt that hip replacement surgery should be reserved for elderly patients. No one knew how long a hip replacement would last. It made sense to only do the operation in older patients whose life expectancy was shorter.

Over time, implant design has improved. Better materials have made the components more durable. Newer techniques for implanting the components have meant that they will stay fixed to bone for a longer period of time. All of these factors mean that a hip replacement is likely to last longer in your body.

Most younger patients want to remain active and will not accept the pain and limitation caused by an arthritic hip. They will not accept the loss of movement of a hip fusion. They do not want to undergo the prolonged recovery and unpredictable results of an osteotomy.

Hip replacement offers predictable relief of pain, a short recovery period, and a low complication rate. For this reason, the number of patients in their 30s, 40s, and 50s having hip replacement surgery is increasing. Some studies show that the number of hip replacement surgeries done in younger patients will soon approach the number being done in the Medicare population.

Newer procedures such as resurfacing arthroplasty conserve bone and are available for younger patients. Alternate **bearing surfaces** (covered later in this book) such as metal on metal and **ceramics** are felt to last longer than traditional metal on polyethylene and are considered an option for younger patients.

The number of patients in their 30s, 40s, and 50s having hip replacement surgery is increasing.

Bearing surfaces

Two surfaces that move against each other in a prosthetic joint.

Ceramic

A hard non-metallic material formed by the action of heat and used as a bearing surface in some hip replacements.

If you are young and contemplating hip replacement surgery, you should remember that you will be placing a higher demand on your new joint than older patients. There will be greater wear over a longer period of time. Even though surgical techniques and materials have improved, it is not yet known what the long-term results will be over a 20-, 30-, or 50-year period. You may need a second surgery or revision procedure years down the line if your first hip wears out.

Before you plan surgery, you should have a frank discussion with your surgeon about the long-term risks and consequences of hip replacement at a young age. You should understand the limits of what you will be able to do in terms of everyday and recreational or sports activities. You will want to do everything possible to make your new hip last as long as it can.

The decision to have hip replacement surgery is a lifetime decision and you want your hip to last a lifetime.

Linda W., a patient, says:

My hips first began to bother me at age 42. I finally went to the doctor. The x-rays showed that I had dysplasia, which contributed to the hip problems I was having. The pain became unbearable, and I knew that I could not live a reasonable life without doing something.

Boris K., a patient, says:

I think it is not a matter of age, but rather a matter of how far the disease has progressed. I asked the doctor all the time, "When should I have surgery?" and the answer always was, "You will feel it yourself." And he was right— when I felt the quality of my life suffer, I decided to go for the surgery.

30. Can I have a total hip replacement if I have had previous hip surgery?

Many patients who are candidates for total hip surgery have had a previous surgical procedure on their hips.

Having surgery on your hip in the past does not prevent you from having a total hip in the future. In fact, many patients have surgery for one problem which leads to arthritis later in life. For example, patients who have had hip disease during childhood or adolescence may function well and have a pain-free hip for many years. They may progress to arthritis as they become older.

Prior surgery may impose special set of circumstances on total hip replacement. The anatomy may be different and there may be scar formation in many areas. The surgeon will try to identify as much of the normal anatomy as possible. He will also try to identify and protect vital structures such as the sciatic nerve, which may be encased in scar and difficult to identify.

Some of the conditions that are often treated surgically prior to total hip replacement are:

1. Developmental Dysplasia of the Hip

   Many infants or children with developmental dysplasia of the hip are treated with **closed reduction** and splinting or bracing. Sometimes an **open reduction** may be necessary. The anatomy of the hip may not be completely normal as it grows. The acetabulum may be more vertical and may have less bone. The femur may be smaller and narrower. The angle of the neck of the femur or *anteversion* may be different than a normal hip. The leg may be shorter than normal.

Closed reduction

A procedure to put a dislocated hip back in place by manipulation.

Open reduction

A procedure to put a dislocated hip back in place by open surgery.

2. Slipped Capital Femoral Epiphysis

Slipped capital femoral epiphysis occurs during the early to mid teenage years. It is often treated by insertion of pins or screws. Sometimes it is necessary to cut the bone to reshape the hip. This is called an *osteotomy*. The osteotomy is held in place with a plate and screws.

If total hip arthroplasty is performed in later years, the fixation hardware may need to be removed. Beyond this, the femoral head and neck may be rounded or deformed. The head may be rotated posteriorly or *retroverted*. All of this will need to be considered if hip replacement is done.

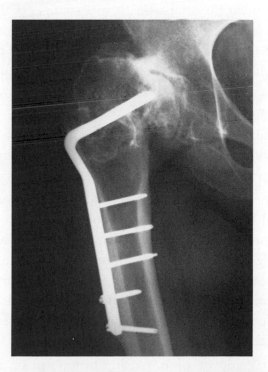

Figure 8   X-ray of patient who had previous osteotomy for SCFE. A plate and screws are present in the femur. The proximal femur is severely deformed. Surgery is more difficult because of the need to remove the hardware and the unusual anatomy.

3. Perthes Disease

Perthes disease is a disease of childhood that occurs between ages 3 and 7 years. Most often treatment is closed and consists of casting or bracing. In teenage years, however, an osteotomy may be performed. As with slipped epiphysis, there may be residual hardware and ongoing deformity of the femoral head and neck.

4. Reconstructive Osteotomy

An osteotomy can also be done as treatment for osteoarthritis in a younger patient. Hardware and scar formation will be a consideration.

5. Hip Fusion

Forty or fifty years ago, hip fusion was done as treatment for osteoarthritis in a younger patient. It was also sometimes done as treatment for an infection of the hip bone or hip joint. In a hip fusion, the cartilage of the femur and the acetabulum has been removed and the bones have been allowed to grow together or fuse.

While hip fusion was frequently successful in relieving pain in younger patients, it completely eliminated any mobility of the hip joint.

Some patients would now like to have the benefits of total hip replacement even though they have had a fusion in the past. The operation is especially difficult because a large amount of bone must be cut, or osteotomized, and removed. Some of the contracted soft tissues around the old joint must be divided. The basic anatomy of the joint must be identified and reestablished.

A "take down" of an old hip fusion can be a difficult procedure, but it is frequently rewarding. Your goals and expectations will play a large role in a decision to have this type of surgery.

6. Post-Traumatic Arthritis

Total hip replacement after fixation for a fracture is common.

A fracture of the femur or acetabulum that has been treated surgically can often lead to post-traumatic arthritis years down the line. Removal of hardware in this situation may make for a bigger operation. If, for example, a rod has been placed in the femur, multiple incisions may have to be made in order to remove all the components of the rod.

By the same token if there has been a surgical repair of the acetabulum, it may be necessary to repeat the acetabular exposure in order to remove all of the hardware that has been placed around the rim of the socket. If the socket has been damaged by the fracture, there may be less bone for placement of the new acetabular component.

7. Avascular Necrosis

Avascular necrosis of the femoral head may be treated primarily with hip replacement, but sometimes a previous surgical procedure has been attempted to prevent collapse of the femoral head. Placement of a cortical bone graft or nail in the neck of the femur will have to be considered when the procedure is planned. The bone graft in the femoral neck may make it more difficult to ream the femoral canal and place a femoral stem.

8. Infection

If you have had previous surgery for an infection in your hip, care has to be taken to make sure that bacteria do not remain within the bone or within the joint. A low grade infection can be present in bone for many years without being obvious clinically.

Your surgeon may want to check for any signs of residual infection before he considers total hip replacement. He will want to take blood tests and may want to do an imaging study such as a bone scan or indium scan. He may even want to withdraw fluid from the joint and send it to the laboratory for culture to make sure there are no bacteria.

During surgery, he may take additional culture specimens and may ask the laboratory to analyze some of the tissue while surgery is still in progress.

Prior infection can make total hip replacement more technically difficult and care should be taken to make sure that none of the infection remains.

In almost all cases, the surgeon is likely to find a large amount of scar tissue if there has been previous surgery.

Your orthopaedic surgeon can discuss any of these conditions with you. He can tell you how your previous hip surgery may affect your upcoming procedure.

31. What is Bipolar (Partial) Hip Replacement?

Bipolar replacement, or arthroplasty, is one type of partial hip replacement that is frequently done for fractures, but can also be done for arthritis, avascular necrosis, and other problems about the hip. It is an option when there is disease of the femoral head, but the acetabulum or socket is not involved. Bipolar arthroplasty provides a way to replace the femoral head without having to ream or put an implant in the socket. It is a more conservative procedure than total hip arthroplasty. In effect, it is a partial hip replacement.

Original partial hip replacements were **unipolar** or **monoblock**. The first of these, designed in 1942 by Dr. Austin Moore, consisted of a large round femoral head attached to a stem which fit inside the normal

Bipolar

A partial hip replacement used to treat fractures and arthritis when the acetabulum is not involved. It consists of a metal stem, a polyethylene inner bearing and a metal outer bearing.

Unipolar

A component that is a single piece with no modular parts. (see also Monoblock)

Monoblock

A component that is a single piece with no modular parts. (see also Unipolar)

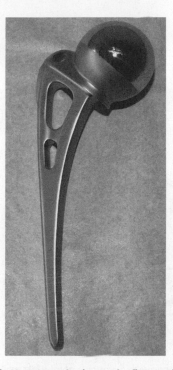

Figure 9   The Austin Moore prosthesis was the first partial hip replacement. It was a single or unipolar replacement with no modular parts.

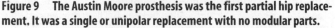

femoral canal. This became known as the *Austin Moore prosthesis* and was a standard in fracture treatment for many years. Later designs updated and refined the concept of a unipolar prosthesis.

It was thought, however, that the large metallic head pressing against the natural articular cartilage of the acetabulum caused excess friction and wear. Many times this led to pain and a less satisfactory result.

The bipolar prosthesis was devised as a way to limit friction and wear against the acetabular surface.

The bipolar prosthesis was first developed by Dr. James Bateman in 1974 in a design he called the *universal proximal femur*. In the past 30 years, the concept of a

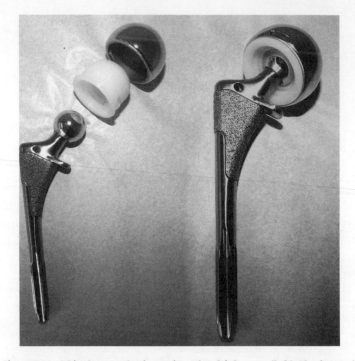

Figure 10   A bipolar prosthesis consists of multiple parts (left). The femoral head and stem are below. The white inner bearing fits over the femoral head. The metal shell or outer bearing snaps onto the inner bearing. An assembled bipolar prosthesis is on the right.

A bipolar prosthesis is a "ball within a ball" or a "head within a head."

Inner bearing

The inner polyethylene layer of a bipolar prosthesis that sits between the femoral head and the outer bearing metal shell.

Outer bearing

The outer metal layer of a bipolar prosthesis that is attached over the inner bearing. The outer bearing makes a joint with the acetabulum.

bipolar prosthesis has been updated and refined by many implant manufacturers.

A bipolar prosthesis is a "ball within a ball" or a "head within a head." It has two mobile articular surfaces rather than one. A small metallic femoral head sits on top of the normal femoral stem. This is the prosthetic femoral head. A second layer, or **inner bearing**, sits on top of the femoral head. The inner bearing is made of the same plastic or polyethylene used in an acetabular component. This creates the same metal on polyethylene bearing surface found in a total hip. An outer metallic shell called the **outer bearing** fits on top of the plastic inner bearing. The outer bearing then articulates with or makes a joint with the normal acetabulum.

Like a unipolar component, the large metallic outer bearing rests against the normal articular cartilage of the socket and in a similar way allows for normal movement of the hip joint.

There is also movement, however, between the small femoral head and the plastic inner bearing surface. Thus there are two layers of movement and two bearing surfaces in bipolar arthroplasty. The addition of a second bearing surface may increase range of motion of the hip, but more importantly it may also reduce the amount of friction and wear on the acetabular side. This will lead to less pain and greater longevity of the prosthesis.

Though multiple studies have been done, it is not clear how much movement occurs at each bearing surface or whether the outer bearing surface becomes fixed in the acetabulum over time.

The diameter of the outer bearing is typically 43 mm or greater and is much larger than the femoral head in a total hip arthroplasty, which is 22–36 mm. For this reason, a bipolar prosthesis tends to be more stable than a standard total hip arthroplasty. It is less likely to dislocate and come out of the joint.

A bipolar arthroplasty has the same femoral stem component as a total hip. It can be converted to a total hip arthroplasty if necessary. Bipolar replacement is most commonly done for fractures. The main indication is a displaced fracture of the femoral neck just below the head of the femur. In this circumstance, the ball of the femur has broken off and is not likely to heal. Accordingly, the treatment is to replace the femoral head with a bipolar prosthesis. This is routinely done for subcapital or femoral neck fractures in elderly patients. A bipolar prosthesis may also be used to treat a femoral neck fracture that has first undergone pinning but then failed to heal.

Bipolar arthroplasty may be done as a primary procedure for problems that cause hip pain but only involve the femoral head. Often this is a young patient with avascular necrosis who has hip pain and collapse of the femoral joint surface but no wear on the acetabulum. In younger patients, this will relieve pain and preserve bone in the socket.

A bipolar prosthesis may also be used for other disease processes such as a bone cyst or tumor, which involve only the femoral head and not the acetabulum.

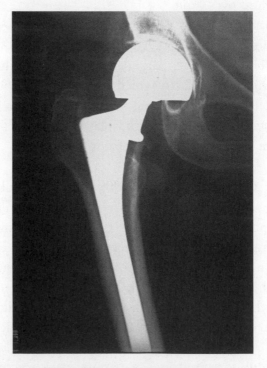

Figure 11   X-ray of a bipolar replacement in a hip joint.

Some of the possible problems of a bipolar prosthesis include groin pain, long-term wear of the acetabular joint cartilage and protrusion of the large metal head into the pelvis. Indeed, some studies show better results for total hip rather than bipolar arthroplasty for reconstructive problems. Other options such as hip resurfacing and limited hip resurfacing are now sometimes used in younger patients.

32. What is resurfacing?

Resurfacing is a type of hip replacement that preserves bone in the proximal femur.

In a standard total hip, the entire femoral head and a large part of the femoral neck are removed and replaced with the femoral component. In resurfacing, only the articular cartilage and the outer portion of the femoral head are removed. The inner portion of the head and the femoral neck are left in place. A cup shaped femoral component is seated over the remaining portion of the femoral head. A small stem extends into part of the femoral neck. In a standard total hip replacement, a much broader and longer femoral stem is inserted well into the proximal shaft of the femur.

Both the femoral and acetabular components are made of a cobalt-chromium metal alloy. Thus, the bearing surfaces are metal on metal. The acetabular component is press fit into the socket. The femoral component is cemented onto the remaining portion of the femoral head. Resurfacing is therefore a **hybrid arthroplasty**.

Resurfacing procedures have been done for approximately 30 years. The initial procedures had metal on polyethylene surfaces and met with limited success.

Hybrid arthroplasty

A joint replacement where one component is cemented in place and the other component is press fit.

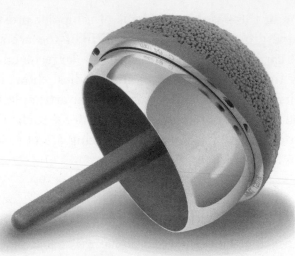

Figure 12   Resurfacing components.

Courtesy of Smith and Nephew.

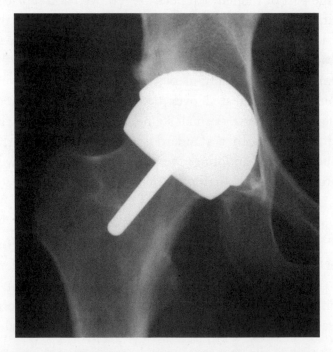

Figure 13   X-ray of resurfacing components. The femoral implant covers the femoral head only and preserves bone in the femoral neck.

Courtesy of Smith and Nephew.

The high failure rate may have been due to polyethylene wear caused by the large diameter femoral component. It was also felt that early failures were due to poor technique.

The demand for a bone sparing procedure in younger patients has led to renewed interest in resurfacing. Better component design and surgical technique have improved results. Ideally, the procedure is performed on a young patient with good bone suffering from either osteoarthritis or post-traumatic arthritis. Adequate bone stock is necessary for the success of the procedure. Patients with a leg length discrepancy are not good candidates. Unlike a conventional total hip, leg lengths cannot be adjusted or corrected by a resurfacing procedure.

Resurfacing has several advantages. The large size femoral head is very stable. Dislocation is a rare event. It is much easier to revise a resurfacing than a standard total hip. If revision is necessary, the femoral head and femoral neck can be removed at the normal level and a conventional femoral stem inserted. The large surface area of the components lessens the risk of impingement on the edge of the acetabulum.

Resurfacing may be a useful option in patients who have a high risk of dislocation, such as those with neurologic disease and poor muscle control. It is also an option for patients with a deformed hip where placement of a standard femoral stem is difficult.

Resurfacing may be done through a standard anterior (front) or posterior (rear) approach to the hip. Since the femoral head is not removed, it must be retracted after it has been dislocated. This requires a longer surgical exposure and more dissection than a conventional total hip. Once the femoral head is exposed, a guide wire is placed at the proper angle through the surface of the head into the femoral neck. A milling or reaming device is placed over the guide wire to shape the femoral head. The acetabular side is reamed and prepared in the same way as a conventional total hip. The all metal acetabular component is impacted into place. The femoral component is cemented onto the remaining surface of the femoral head. The joint is then reduced and checked for alignment and stability.

Resurfacing is best done in young patients with good bone and a normal shaped femoral head. Patients who should not have the procedure are patients with:

- osteoporosis
- poor bone quality in the femoral head or femoral neck
- metabolic bone disease
- avascular necrosis with femoral head collapse
- large degenerative cysts in the femoral head or femoral neck

The procedure is also not ideal for patients who are overweight, have abnormal metal sensitivity, or have kidney problems. It is not known if the kidneys are affected by the metallic ion particles given off by wear of the metal on metal bearing. Resurfacing is also difficult in patients such as those who have had Perthes disease in childhood and have residual deformities of the femoral head and neck.

Recent studies have shown that with modern surgical technique and good patient selection, short-term clinical success rates have been high. Since the procedure is relatively new, long-term results and survivorship are not yet available.

The most common cause for revision of a resurfacing procedure is femoral neck fracture. This usually occurs in the first few months after surgery and may be technique dependent. In some cases, a fracture of the femoral neck may be treated by limited weight bearing and no surgery. Most of the time, conversion to a conventional total hip is required. Studies show the incidence of femoral neck fracture following resurfacing to be in the range of 1% to 1.5%.

Limited resurfacing is one more option for younger patients. In limited resurfacing, only the femoral component is applied. The acetabulum is left untouched. This can be done if the hip disease involves the femoral head only and there are no degenerative changes in the acetabulum. While this preserves the acetabulum, patients may sometimes complain of groin pain. This is caused by pressure of the metal femoral head on the native articular cartilage of the socket.

Limited resurfacing
A resurfacing procedure where only the femoral component is applied. This can be done if the hip disease involves only the femoral head and not the acetabulum.

Hip resurfacing is gaining in popularity. As more procedures are done, techniques will improve, and we will have a greater understanding of the long-term survivorship and complications.

33. What is a hip fusion?

A hip fusion is a procedure where the ball of the femur and socket are brought together to form a single bone. The purpose of the fusion is to relieve pain and to stabilize the hip joint.

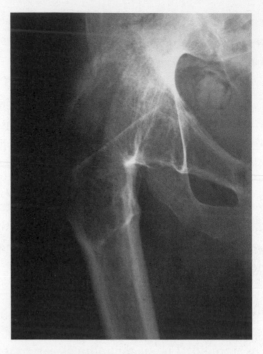

Figure 14   X-ray of a hip that has been fused for over fifty years. The femur has been joined to the pelvis to form a single long continuous bone.

In a hip fusion, the articular cartilage on the two joint surfaces is removed. This exposes raw cancellous bone with good surfaces for healing. When the cartilage is removed and the bones are put together, the two bone surfaces will heal to one another and form a single unit. The bones are thus fused together. The technical name for this procedure is **hip arthrodesis**.

Fusing the bones together relieves the pain of an arthritic hip. It also stabilizes the joint. When the hip has been fused, the results are permanent. The down side is that even though a fusion relieves pain, it eliminates all motion at the hip joint. A person with a hip fusion will never again be able to move the joint or to have a normal gait.

Hip arthrodesis
Surgical fusion of the ball and socket of the hip joint to form one continuous bone.

When the hip has been fused, the results are permanent.

Hip fusion was first performed in the early part of the 20th century. For many years it was a standard treatment for painful osteoarthritis of the hip. With the advent of cup arthroplasty in the 1940s and total hip arthroplasty in the late 1960s, hip fusion has become less popular. Originally, it was felt that the best patient for a hip fusion was an active individual younger than forty years of age with arthritis in a single hip. A hip fusion puts additional stress on the opposite hip, the lumbar spine, and the knee on the same side. It was not appropriate for patients with problems in these areas. Most hip fusion patients were young and had arthritis due to previous fracture or an old infection.

The success of total hip arthroplasty has made hip fusion less desirable, even for patients in their twenties and thirties. Younger active patients who have total hip arthroplasty know that they may need a revision procedure when they get older. Despite this, most will not accept the loss of mobility, abnormal gait, and prolonged recovery time that come with a hip fusion.

Hip fusion is done through a long incision on the front or anterior aspect of the hip joint. The joint capsule is incised and the hip joint is exposed. All of the articular cartilage is removed from both sides of the joint. The bones are then shaped to fit together. Internal fixation with screws or a metal plate and screws is used to hold the fusion together. Bone graft material may be placed around the fusion to add additional bony surface and to speed the healing.

The hip is fused in a slightly bent or flexed position and a position of slight external rotation. Care is taken to allow enough flexion for sitting but not to flex the hip too much so that the leg is very shortened. This will allow the best position for daily function and activities.

Years ago patients were placed in *spica* cast from the waist to the toes of the surgical leg after the procedure. Modern methods of internal fixation, however, are much stronger and most patients do not need a cast. A period of nonweight bearing or partial weight bearing on crutches is required until healing is complete. The progress of the fusion and the degree of healing can be assessed with periodic x-rays.

A patient may be full weight bearing once the fusion has completely healed. This may take 3 to 6 months.

Nonunion or failure of the fusion to heal is the major complication of the procedure. With modern techniques, this occurs in about 10–15% of patients. If nonunion occurs, a repeat fusion needs to be done. As with any surgical procedure, infection can also be a complication.

Hip fusion puts additional strain on the joints surrounding the hip. It may put pressure on the lumbar spine or cause pain in the knee joint below the hip. Beyond this, it may affect the opposite hip. This is because patients must compensate for the loss of motion in the fused hip joint. Individuals with pain in these areas or a disease such as rheumatoid arthritis that involves multiple joints are not candidates for hip fusion.

In some circumstances, hip fusion is still used as a salvage procedure following an infected total hip arthroplasty.

The popularity of total hip arthroplasty has led many patients who have had hip fusion to seek conversion to a total hip. They would like to regain the mobility that was lost when their hip was fused.

Conversion of a fusion to a total hip can be a technically demanding procedure. Since the joint surfaces are fused together, they must first be separated at the appropriate level and the bones reshaped to accept the prosthetic components. The anatomy is distorted and accurate component placement is more difficult. While the results of a fusion takedown and conversion to arthroplasty may be gratifying, the overall incidence of complications is higher than that for primary total hip arthroplasty. Even though hip fusion provides a durable long-term solution for painful hip, most younger patients will not accept the limitations of function and motion that come with fusion. Since total hip arthroplasty has become so popular, hip fusions are now relatively rare.

34. What is an osteotomy?

Osteotomy literally means *cutting of the bone.*

In orthopaedic surgery, an osteotomy is an operation where a section of the bone is cut so that the bone may be realigned to a better position. An osteotomy can change the angle or the rotation of a bone which, in turn, can affect the function of a nearby joint. In the hip, this is done to relieve pressure on the arthritic surface of a joint. The two most common indications for osteotomy of the hip are osteoarthritis and avascular necrosis. The goal is to transfer weight bearing from an area of diseased cartilage to an area of normal cartilage.

By making a cut in the proximal femur just below the joint, the joint surface or articular surface of the femoral head can be rotated so that normal cartilage is placed in the position of greatest stress. While this will not cure the underlying arthritis or avascular necrosis, it may buy time in a younger patient and delay the need for hip replacement surgery.

An operation that increases the angle of the hip is called a *valgus osteotomy*; an operation that decreases the angle of the hip is called a *varus osteotomy*.

Sometimes the hip joint socket or acetabulum is too shallow and there is no covering over part of the femoral head. In this case, a cut through the bone of the pelvis or *pelvic osteotomy* may be done to slide bone over the uncovered femoral head.

As part of an osteotomy, bone may be removed or bone graft may be added to the femur. In rare circumstances, both pelvic and femoral osteotomies may be done if there are deformities on both sides of the hip joint.

The surgeon will take measurements from preoperative x-rays and CT scan to determine the exact angle of the cut. He will try to rotate the bone so that the normal articular surface is placed in a position of comfort for the patient. An osteotomy requires some form of internal fixation such as plates and screws to hold the two parts of the bone together while healing takes place. Most often there will be a period of limited or protected weight bearing after surgery.

An osteotomy is a procedure to buy time in a younger patient who wants to preserve his or her natural hip for as long as possible.

As noted, an osteotomy is a procedure to buy time in a younger patient who wants to preserve his or her natural hip for as long as possible. Most surgeons recognize, however, that a total hip replacement may be necessary years down the line. For this reason, care is taken to make sure that the hip is aligned in a way that does not interfere with placement of total hip components.

35. What is core decompression?

Core decompression is a surgical procedure used to treat hip pain in the early stages of avascular necrosis.

One of the causes of pain in AVN is increased pressure in the bone marrow of the diseased portion of the femoral head. Reducing the pressure in this area may relieve the pain of AVN and allow healing to take place.

Core decompression involves drilling of the femoral neck and femoral head. Drilling of the diseased area reduces pressure in the small vessels of the bone marrow. This allows for greater blood flow and promotes healing of the bone. The procedure can be done under spinal or **general anesthesia**. The patient is placed in the supine or lying down position on a fracture table. A special x-ray machine called an *image intensifier* provides either intermittent or continuous x-ray in several planes. In this way, the exact area of necrosis can be identified and the position of the instruments can be followed during the course of the procedure.

After a skin incision is made, a guide wire is passed from the side of the hip in to the diseased portion of the femoral head. The location of the guide wire is checked with the image intensifier. When this is satisfactory, a channel is made over the wire with a larger drill. This will drill out the zone of necrosis and relieve pressure in the area. The surgeon may choose to fill the defect with bone graft material. Some grafts are vascularized and have a blood supply from an adjacent area. An alternate procedure is to place a small nail within the femoral neck to support the bone while it is healing.

Core decompression can only be done in the early stages of avascular necrosis. At this point there is pain but little loss of motion. The changes may be seen only on an MRI study and not a plain x-ray. The joint surface of the femur should remain smooth and round. If the joint surface has collapsed it means the disease is

General anesthesia
Anesthesia where a patient is put to sleep and is completely unconscious.

more advanced. When this happens, core decompression is not likely to be successful in relieving pain.

Since the procedure requires removal of bone, many surgeons will recommend a period of partial or non-weight bearing with crutches for 6 to 12 weeks until the hip has fully healed. This may have to be modified if surgery is done on both sides.

Core decompression can relieve the pain of avascular necrosis in early stages. It may help to preserve the normal femoral head and be an alternative to hip replacement.

36. Is there a role for arthroscopy?

Arthroscopy is being used more and more for treatment of a painful hip. While arthroscopic procedures are most commonly done in the knee, shoulder and elbow, more surgeons are gaining experience with arthroscopy of the hip.

Arthroscopy is a technique that uses a fiberoptic scope and small instruments to perform surgery on a joint.

Arthroscopy is a technique that uses a fiberoptic scope and small instruments to perform surgery on a joint. The scope and instruments are inserted through three or four tiny incisions called *portals*. A light source and a television camera are connected to the arthroscope. The surgeon then views the inside of the hip joint on a television monitor as he uses his instruments to do the procedure.

The procedure is done under general anesthesia. Most often the patient is lying on his side with the operative side facing up towards the surgeon. This is called the *lateral decubitus position*. The procedure can also be performed with the patient lying flat or supine. Traction is applied to the leg to separate the joint surfaces and create a wider space to place the arthroscope and instruments.

Arthroscopy may be used as both a diagnostic and therapeutic procedure in the hip. It can be used to evaluate the cause of a painful hip when plain x-rays and MRI have been negative. It may identify a problem causing mechanical symptoms such as clicking, snapping, or catching in the joint. Surgery can then be done to treat the problem under arthroscopic control.

Some of the problems treated by hip arthroscopy include removal of free fragments of bone or cartilage called **loose bodies** and removal of arthritic bone spurs called osteophytes. The osteophytes may impinge on the edge of the joint and cause mechanical symptoms.

Loose bodies
Free fragments of bone or cartilage within a joint.

In one condition, **synovial chondromatosis**, multiple loose bodies form from articular cartilage. These cannot be seen on a plain x-ray and sometimes are not completely visible on MRI. The loose bodies cause pain and catching within the joint.

Synovial chondromatosis
A condition where multiple loose bodies form in the joint from articular cartilage.

In the past, treatment of synovial chondromatosis of the hip was by an open incision or arthrotomy. Now the procedure can be done with much less trauma arthroscopically.

A tear of the ligament surrounding the hip joint, the *acetabular labrum*, can sometimes be repaired arthroscopically. If the labrum breaks off and tears, the loose fragment may cause pain, catching, and mechanical clunking within the joint. This fragment may be removed arthroscopically or sutured back in place by advanced techniques.

Arthroscopy may diagnose an early case of osteoarthritis even though other studies are negative. Scuffing or damage to the articular surface seen through an arthroscope may be the cause of pain in the groin and thigh. In more advanced cases, a shaving or smoothing of the painful joint surfaces called an *arthroscopic debridement* or *chondroplasty* may be done. The long-term benefits of this type of procedure, however, are not clear.

Arthroscopy may be helpful in assessing the joint surface in a hip with avascular necrosis. Some surgical procedures for the treatment of AVN require that the joint surface be smooth and intact. These are procedures such as core decompression or bone grafting that are normally done before the femoral joint surface collapses. If the joint surface is collapsed then the treatment would be arthroplasty or replacement. In this situation, arthroscopy can be used to determine the status of the joint and whether or not a joint preserving procedure will be effective.

Finally, arthroscopy can be useful as a diagnostic procedure in a painful or infected total hip. An arthroscopic drainage can be done if the joint is infected.

Arthroscopy is done as an outpatient surgical procedure under general anesthesia. Most patients will be on crutches for a period of time to protect the joint after surgery. Sutures are removed 7 to 10 days postoperatively. The physical therapy and rehabilitation program is determined by the operating surgeon based upon the findings. It may be several months before a patient is able to return to sports.

Known complications of arthroscopy include bruising or injury to the articular surface by the scope and temporary nerve palsy resulting from traction applied during surgery. Most complications are temporary and resolve quickly with treatment.

Arthroscopy is evolving as a technique. More surgeons are learning to do the procedure and better instruments are being developed. It is likely that arthroscopy will play a greater role in the future in the diagnosis and treatment of a painful hip.

PART SEVEN

The Operation— Total Hip Replacement

How can I prepare for surgery?

Who will do the surgery?

How is the surgery done?

More . . .

37. How can I prepare for surgery?

Once you have decided to have total hip surgery it is important to plan for your procedure and your care after surgery. It is helpful to involve your family or caregivers in the planning process.

First you will arrange a date for surgery with your doctor's office. Most surgeons have 1 or 2 specific days during the week when they do surgery. Elective hip surgery is scheduled several weeks in advance. This gives you and your family time to prepare.

Elective hip surgery is scheduled several weeks in advance. This gives you and your family time to prepare.

Many hospitals now offer preoperative teaching classes for total joint patients. You will meet some of the nursing staff and get information about your care in the hospital. They will tell you what to bring (pajamas, slippers etc.), where you will stay, and when is the best time for visitors. They will explain physical therapy and give you information about the discharge planning process.

Your doctor may also provide booklets or written information about the procedure. If you have a computer, he may direct you to articles on the internet. Try to find out as much as you can about the procedure and what you can expect after surgery.

You will need to have testing before surgery to make sure that it is safe for you to have anesthesia and the surgical procedure. Typically this consists of blood tests, chest x-ray, electrocardiogram, and urinalysis. Your doctor's office will help you schedule a time and place for your testing.

Your surgeon may recommend that you see your family physician or internist for a preoperative medical evaluation. This is to make sure that you are medically cleared to have anesthesia and surgery.

He may also ask you to bathe the skin around your hip with an antiseptic soap on the day before you come to the hospital.

Finally, your surgeon's office will tell you when and where you need to arrive at the hospital on the day of surgery.

You should not eat or drink anything by mouth after midnight on the night before surgery unless your doctor tells you to take your normal medicines with a sip of water.

Linda C., a patient, says:

I had known for several years that hip replacement would be necessary. I prepared for the surgery beforehand by doing exercises and losing twenty pounds.

Cheley H., an Orthopaedic Head Nurse, says:

For many years, I have had the great fortune to be able to teach a preoperative total joint replacement class to patients scheduled to receive new hips or knees. Education encourages patients to become active participants in their own plan of care. At times, patients are uncertain about the decision to have surgery. The only regret I have ever heard from a recovered joint replacement patient is "I wish that I hadn't waited so long."

38. Should I see my regular doctor before surgery?

Your orthopaedic surgeon may ask that you have a general medical checkup before you come in to the hospital. The place to start is with your regular physician. Usually, this is a physician who specializes in internal medicine or family practice. He or she will have a good knowledge of general medicine and will identify any medical problems that need to be addressed before surgery.

If you do not have a family physician, your orthopaedic surgeon may be able to provide a referral.

Your internist or family practitioner will do a medical clearance. He will review your medical history, physical examination, and your preoperative testing and will order any additional tests that need to be done. He will determine if any medical problems require further evaluation before surgery. If you are taking certain medications, he will tell you what medications need to be taken on the day of surgery or if any medications need to be stopped.

If you are taking certain medications, he will tell you what medications need to be taken on the day of surgery or if any medications need to be stopped.

For example, if you are on a maintenance dose of steroid medication such as Prednisone, your doctor will make sure that you are given the proper doses before surgery and that the medication is continued afterward. If you are diabetic and take insulin, you will need to know what dose to take on the morning of surgery and what dose to take afterward. Your insulin dose is likely to increase in the postoperative period due to the stress of surgery.

If you are on a blood thinner, such as Coumadin, your internist or family physician will tell you when to stop taking the medication. For some heart problems, it may be necessary for you to have some kind of anticoagulation until right before the day of surgery. When you stop Coumadin you will go on a blood thinner with a shorter duration of activity such as Lovenox.

This can be taken up until a few hours before surgery. Your primary physician will regulate the timing and dosage of any anticoagulation before you go to the operating room. During this period, he may want to obtain blood tests to monitor your status.

Your regular physician can refer you to a subspecialist if you have certain types of medical problems. If you have heart disease, he may ask you to see a cardiologist to evaluate your cardiac status. The cardiologist could do further cardiac testing such as an echocardiogram or stress test. He would also determine if you needed special monitoring such as telemetry after surgery.

If you have a history of asthma or chronic lung disease, your regular physician may ask that you see a pulmonologist so that the condition of your lungs is optimized before you have anesthesia.

He might also refer you to a urologist if you have chronic urinary problems that could cause an infection.

If a serious medical problem is identified, you may have to delay or postpone surgery until the problem can be treated. While this can be frustrating, it is better not to have a problem in the operating room or in the hospital after surgery.

When you are in the hospital, your regular physician may visit you or designate a hospital based physician called a *hospitalist* to see you in his place.

Overall, most people will require preoperative medical clearance before surgery. If you are young, healthy, and have no ongoing health issues or medical problems, then a medical consultation may not be necessary. If there is any question, you should ask your orthopaedic surgeon whether you need clearance at the time you schedule your surgery.

39. Should I donate blood before surgery? Can my friends and family donate blood?

Many patients undergoing total hip arthroplasty will require transfusion either during surgery or in the postoperative period. For this reason, you may choose to donate your own blood in the weeks before surgery in case a transfusion is necessary.

The process by which you donate blood for surgery is called *autologous blood donation*. You donate your own blood to the blood bank at the hospital where you are having surgery. The blood can be stored for about 5 weeks. Most patients will donate a first unit two and a half weeks before the scheduled day of surgery and the second unit one and a half weeks before surgery. Maintaining a time interval between blood donation and surgery will allow your body to form new blood cells and rebuild your blood count after donation. You may be given medication such as iron to help your body form new red blood cells.

The blood you have given is processed by the blood bank and will be available during surgery and afterwards. Most patients who are in good general health are candidates for autologous blood donation. If, however, you have a low blood count, chronic anemia or other medical condition where blood donation might put you at risk, then autologous blood donation should not be considered. Your orthopaedic surgeon and your primary physician can help you make this decision.

The obvious benefit of donating your own blood is that you are not exposed to diseases such as hepatitis and HIV, which may in very rare instances be transmitted through banked blood. Even though the risks of transmission through banked blood are very small, they are not zero.

It is not known what percentage of donated autologous blood is actually given back to patients undergoing hip surgery. In some circumstances you may give blood but not require transfusion at all.

If you cannot give your own blood then directed blood donation from a relative or friend may be an option. Of course, the blood would have to be compatible with your own blood type in order to be useful.

Interestingly enough, using directed blood does not appear to lessen the risks of disease transmission as compared to banked blood.

Options are also available for blood collection during and after surgery. Most commonly a suction drain is used that can store blood for up to six hours after surgery. The blood can then be given back as a transfusion as soon as it has been collected.

Most patients will choose to give their own blood or have directed blood given before surgery. Your orthopaedic surgeon can review your blood donation options with you.

40. What kind of anesthesia will I have?

If you are having surgery you will need to have anesthesia. Anesthesia means *without feeling*. For hip replacement surgery, anesthesia can be either general or regional.

With general anesthesia, you are completely asleep. Regional anesthesia means you are awake but the lower part of your body is numb and you can't feel any pain. Each has its advantages.

The doctor who gives you anesthesia is an *anesthesiologist*. An anesthesiologist specializes in relief of pain and administration of anesthesia to surgical patients. He or she does at least four years of training after medical school. One year is general medicine or surgery. The next three years are spent in an anesthesia residency. Many anesthesiologists also choose to do an additional year of fellowship in one area.

The anesthesiologist may be assisted during the procedure by a nurse anesthetist known as a CRNA.

You will meet the anesthesiologist in the preoperative area before surgery. He will ask questions about your medical history. He will want to know if you have had anesthesia before or if you or anyone in your family has had problems with anesthesia in the past. He will want to know the medications you are taking and if you have any allergies. He will also do a brief examination and review your laboratory tests.

An intravenous line or IV will be started in the preop area. You may be given some medication before you go into the operating room.

In the operating room, the anesthesiologist will attach small devices to your arms and chest before he begins anesthesia. These instruments monitor your blood pressure, heart rate, electrocardiogram and the amount of oxygen in your body.

There are three main types of anesthesia for hip replacement surgery:

- general
- spinal
- epidural

With general anesthesia, you are put to sleep and you are completely unconscious. The anesthesiologist first gives medication to put you to sleep through the IV line. He will then place a device into the back of your throat or into your windpipe, This opens a channel to allow air and anesthesia gases to move directly into your lungs.

The device he places is either an *endotracheal tube* or an *LMA*. An endotracheal tube has been the standard in general anesthesia for many years. It is a tube placed into your windpipe or trachea to maintain a direct airway to your lungs. LMA or laryngeal mask airway is a small mask inserted in back of the throat instead of the trachea. It has been used in the United States for 15 years. Use of an LMA means you are less likely to have a sore throat that can result from an endotracheal tube. The anesthesiologist will assist you with breathing while the ET tube or LMA is in place.

Spinal and **epidural** are *regional anaesthesia*. You are given an injection with medication in your lower spine. Your body loses feeling below the level of injection. You are given some sedation as well as oxygen during the surgery.

Spinal anesthesia is single injection placed inside the lining that surrounds the spinal cord. It can provide anesthesia for several hours. The medication given is

Spinal

Regional anesthesia given by a single injection placed inside the lining that surrounds the spinal cord.

Epidural

Regional anesthesia given by a small catheter placed outside the lining of the spinal cord.

usually morphine, a local anesthetic, or a combination of both.

Epidural anesthesia is a small catheter placed outside the lining of the spinal cord. Medication flows through the catheter. The catheter may be left in place for 1 or 2 days after surgery to help control pain in the postoperative period. Epidural anesthesia is familiar to many women as it is often used during childbirth.

After the procedure you will be taken to a recovery room, or PACU (Post Anesthesia Care Unit). You will remain there until you are completely awake or reacted, your vital signs are stable and you are ready to return to a regular hospital room.

41. Who will do the surgery?

Hip replacement surgery is done by an orthopaedic surgeon. An orthopaedic surgeon is a physician trained in the care of problems and diseases of the musculoskeletal system.

An orthopaedic surgeon is a physician trained in the care of problems and diseases of the musculoskeletal system.

The term *orthopaedic* was first used by Nicholas Andry, a professor of medicine at the University of Paris. It is derived from Greek words, which literally mean *straight child*. In 1741, Andry published a book called *Orthopaedia or the Art of Correcting and Preventing Deformities in Children*. Since that time the term orthopaedic has come in to common use to describe physicians and surgeons who take care of musculoskeletal problems.

While the primary focus of orthopaedic care is bones, orthopaedic surgeons treat disease of structures around the bones as well. These include joints, muscles, tendons, ligaments, and nerves.

It takes a long time to become an orthopaedic surgeon. At the start, an orthopaedic surgeon goes to college for 4 years to earn his bachelors degree. He or she then goes on for another 4 years to an accredited medical school. After graduating medical school, a physician can be licensed to practice but does not have training in any specialty.

Most orthopaedic surgeons do 5 years of residency. The term *resident* came about because years ago most doctors in training lived at the hospital where they worked. Now residents often rotate through several hospitals as part of an orthopaedic residency program. As a rule, they sleep in the hospital only on nights when they take call.

The first year consists of training in general surgery and surgical related fields or subspecialties. This includes both learning how to do surgery and taking care of hospital patients with surgical diseases.

For the next four years, training is mainly in orthopaedic surgery. There are rotations through many different areas of orthopaedic surgery, including fractures and trauma, pediatric problems, hand, sports medicine, foot and ankle, shoulder and elbow, arthroscopy, tumors, and joint replacement. Training involves not only surgery but caring for sick hospital patients, outpatient clinics, and rehabilitation following orthopaedic surgery.

Some residents spend extra time during their training doing laboratory research.

After residency, surgeons may take an additional year of fellowship at another hospital or university in a specific area such as joint replacement, trauma, or sports medicine.

Most orthopaedic surgeons become *board certified*. An orthopaedic surgeon who is board certified is a Diplomate of the American Board of Orthopaedic Surgery. This is one of twenty-four subspecialty boards under the American Board of Medical Specialties. Surgeons who have passed board requirements have met a high standard of subspecialty qualification. Certification is not a license but many hospitals make board certification a requirement for maintaining hospital privileges.

In order to be board certified, an orthopaedic surgeon must first pass a written exam, then an oral examination which can be taken only after 22 months of clinical practice. Certification is also based on recommendations from fellow orthopaedic surgeons, department chairman, and hospital chiefs of staff.

Board certification is a time-limited process. Orthopaedic surgeons must re-certify every 10 years.

After certification, an orthopaedic surgeon may become a Fellow of the American Academy of Orthopaedic Surgeons.

Osteopathic physicians may be certified by the American Osteopathic Board of Orthopaedic Surgery.

42. Who else will be in the operating room?

In the operating room, an orthopaedic surgeon doing hip replacement will have one or two assistants at the operating table. The assistant may be another orthopaedic surgeon, a physician's assistant (PA) or registered nurse first assistant (RNFA). Both PAs and RNFAs are trained to work with surgeons in the operating room as first assistants.

A scrub nurse will also be in the sterile operating field with the surgeons. The scrub nurse may be a registered nurse, licensed practical nurse, or certified scrub technician. The job of the scrub nurse is to pass the surgical tools and instruments to the surgeon and to keep track of all of the instruments and equipment within the sterile field. A circulating nurse, or circulator, is in the operating room but is not scrubbed in to the procedure. The circulator retrieves and opens sterile equipment, takes care of the medical record, answers the phone, and does everything in the operating room necessary to move the case along.

In joint replacement cases, the circulator opens the packaging of the specific joint replacement components and passes them in a sterile manner to the scrub nurse.

In some operating rooms, a representative of the implant manufacturer may be present during joint replacement cases. He is not scrubbed and is not at the operating table. His purpose is to make sure that the right instruments for the implant are available and to make sure the proper components are opened.

43. How is the surgery done?

Surgery is done with the patient either lying down (supine) or on his or her side (lateral decubitus). Several surgical approaches can be made—anterior (from the front), posterior (from the back) or approaches closer to the side—anterolateral, posterolateral.

An incision is made through the skin and the fat layer beneath the skin. Depending on the approach, the muscles either in front or back of the hip are separated so that an interval or plane can be created that will lead to the joint. Sometimes some of the smaller muscles need to be divided in order to reach the joint. If surgery is by a posterior approach the sciatic nerve is identified so that it may be protected during the procedure.

The lining of the joint, the capsule, is exposed and an incision is made. At this point, joint fluid or synovial fluid usually extrudes from the joint. When the capsule is divided the hip joint can be seen. The femoral head can be visualized within the socket. The leg is then rotated so that the head of the femur is dislocated or comes out of the socket. If surgery is being done for arthritis the damage to the articular cartilage, the surface of the joint, is evident.

The neck of the femur below the femoral head is exposed. A saw is then used to cut the neck of the femur so that the femoral head can be removed. Sometimes the neck of the femur is cut when the femoral head is still in the acetabulum. The head is then removed from the socket after the neck is cut. Once the femoral head has been removed, the remaining part of the femoral neck can be retracted so that the joint surface of the acetabulum is exposed. Arthritic changes, if present, are visible in the socket as well.

The soft tissue lining around the rim of the socket, the *labrum,* is removed. The socket is then prepared to receive the acetabular component of the hip replacement. The remaining joint cartilage is removed and the acetabulum is prepared by round or spherical power driven reamers. The reamers remove some of the bone beneath the surface to create room for the implant. Reaming is begun with a small diameter reamer. The reamers are then increased in size by one or two millimeters until there is a good tight fit of the reamer in the socket. An acetabular component may then be placed that is the same size as the reamer or one to two millimeters larger. This will insure that the component fits tightly.

The outer metal shell of the acetabular component can then be driven or impacted into place in the prepared socket. If there is a tight fit it may be left alone. If the component does not feel completely secure, one or two screws may be inserted through holes in the metal shell into the bone of the pelvis. Once the metal shell is impacted and fixed in the bone, the polyethylene liner that fits inside the metal shell is placed. If the component is to be cemented, then the cement is mixed and pressed into the prepared socket. The component is then positioned inside the cement. Pressure is then maintained on the component until the cement is dry so that the position does not change.

The acetabular side of the joint replacement is complete. The surgeon can now begin to work on the femur. The neck of the femur is then brought back into the surgical field and retractors are positioned.

A surgical drill or an awl is then used to identify the canal of the femur which will receive the stem of the femoral component. Once the canal has been opened it may be widened with reamers in $1/2$ to one millimeter increments. A special orthopaedic chisel called a **rasp** or *broach* is then used to carve a space in the area below the femoral neck called the **metaphysis**. The rasp has the same shape as the actual femoral component and can be used as a trial component before the permanent component is implanted. Next, a trial femoral head and neck component is put on top of the rasp. The diameter of the head matches the diameter of the polyethylene liner of the socket. The neck lengths

Rasp

A special orthopaedic chisel used to prepare the medullary canal of the femur.

Metaphysis

A wide area of the femur between the femoral neck and shaft of the bone.

come in different sizes so that the surgeon can restore the joint to its proper height.

Once the trial components are positioned, the ball is put into the socket and the joint is tested. This is called a **trial reduction**. The surgeon moves the hip in several directions to make sure the joint stays in place and the ball does not come out of the socket. He also checks to see if the joint is too loose or too tight and to make sure that the length of both legs is equal. If there is a problem, he can make adjustments.

The trial femoral head and the rasp are removed. The permanent stem is driven into place or cemented in the femoral canal. The head and neck component is seated on the stem.

At this point, the field is checked to make sure that no loose pieces of bone or tissue are sitting in the socket. The hip joint is then permanently put into place or reduced. It is once more tested through a range of motion. The wound is washed out or *irrigated* with a saline solution and is checked to make sure there is no active bleeding. A drainage tube may be placed deep in the wound and brought through a separate small skin puncture away from the incision. The tube is connected to an external suction drain and is removed the day after surgery. The deep muscle layers in the wound are closed together with sutures. The layer of fat or *fascia* beneath the skin is also closed. The skin edges are brought together either with sutures or small metal staples.

At the end of the procedure a dressing is applied to the wound. The patient is awakened if he or she has had general anesthesia. He is then transferred to a bed or

Trial reduction

Part of a hip replacement procedure where trial components are inserted and the femoral head is placed in the socket. The joint is then checked for alignment and stability before permanent components are inserted.

stretcher. A hip *abduction pillow* may be placed between the legs to prevent them from crossing and causing a dislocation. A skin traction boot may also be applied for this purpose. When the patient is safely awakened from anesthesia he is taken to the recovery room area on the bed or stretcher.

44. How long does the procedure take to perform?

It takes most surgeons between 1 and 2 hours to perform a routine total hip replacement. Not all of the time spent in the operating room, however, is taken up by the surgery itself.

You will first be brought to the operating room in a bed or on a stretcher, then transfer to the operating table. The anesthesiologist will start an intravenous line and attach monitors for an electrocardiogram, for blood pressure, and for the amount of oxygen in your blood.

The anesthesiologist will check to make sure that your initial readings are stable before he begins anesthesia.

It may take several minutes to put you to sleep, or longer if you are having a spinal or epidural anesthetic.

The operating team will check to make sure that the correct side has been identified, note any allergies, metal implants, or other relevant information.

Once you are asleep, it takes additional time to position you on the operating table. The anesthesiologist, surgeon, and operating team will check to make sure that you are properly secured and all potential pressure areas are padded.

Your leg, hip, and thigh will then be scrubbed and prepped with an antiseptic solution. This is typically iodine based, but other solutions may be used if you have an allergy to iodine. When this has been done, sterile drapes will be placed to isolate this surgical field.

It may be 15 to 30 minutes from the time you come to the operating room till the time the procedure actually starts.

When surgery is completed, a sterile dressing will be applied over the wound. If a drain has been placed in the wound, it will be connected to an outside pump or container. Additional time is needed to come out of anesthesia.

Once anesthesia is finished you will be transferred to a bed. An abduction pillow or skin traction may be placed on your leg to prevent dislocation. At the end of the procedure, you will be taken to a post-anesthesia or recovery room area.

All told your time in the operating room may last from 1 to 3 hours for a routine total hip.

45. What are the components made of?

Most hip replacements are made up of a combination of metal and plastic.

Most hip replacements are made up of a combination of metal and plastic. The femoral head and femoral stem are metal. The acetabular component is a durable plastic. Together, these materials work together to create a strong joint that moves smoothly as you sit, stand and walk. There is very little friction as the ball moves inside the socket.

The two surfaces that rub against each other inside the joint are called *bearing surfaces*. The most common bearing surfaces are metal on polyethylene.

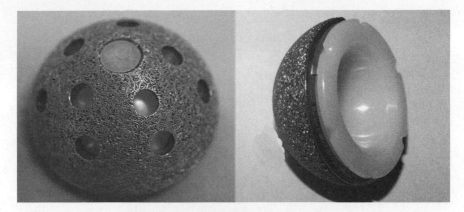

Figure 15 Outer titantium metal shell of an acetabular component with a porous surface is seen on the left. Picture at right shows the metal shell with the inner polyethylene liner.

The metals used for both the femoral head bearing sur face and the femoral stem are alloys such as stainless steel, cobalt-chromium, and titanium. Alloys are a combination of metals that are put together for maximum strength. Ideally, metal that is used in a hip replacement should be inert, corrosion resistant, nonmagnetic and biocompatible. It should have good longevity and be resistant to bending or breakage.

The first femoral components designed by Charnley were stainless steel. Now most components are made of cobalt-chromium and titanium. Cobalt-chromium and titanium have a longer fatigue life than stainless steel. They are also more adaptable to having porous surfaces, which are now used with bone ingrowth components.

Cobalt-chromium is the best metal for the bearing surface of the femoral head. It is relatively resistant to wear and to corrosion. It is less likely to breakdown at the surface. Titanium is a better alloy for a femoral stem because its elastic properties are closer to those of bone. Most modular components now have a cobalt-chromium head and a titanium stem.

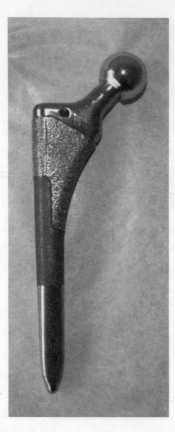

Figure 16   A femoral component with a cobalt-chromium head and a titanium stem.

The bearing surface for the socket or acetabulum is ultra high molecular weight polyethylene (UHMWPE), a strong plastic that is chemically inert. Polyethylene is a widely used plastic. It is a polymer made up of repeating units of ethylene chemically bonded together. UHMWPE is an especially durable polyethylene made up of large molecules. It has good resistance to deformity or *creep* but does give off some wear particles into the hip joint.

The first acetabular components were completely polyethylene and made to be implanted with cement. Most acetabular components are now a combination of an inner UHMWPE liner and an outer metal shell.

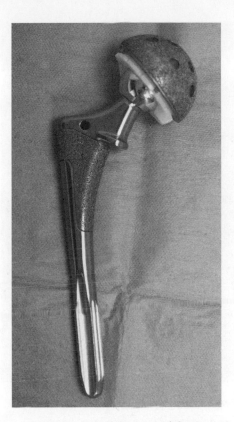

Figure 17 Femoral and acetabular components joined together as a total hip arthroplasty.

© American Academy of Orthopaedic Surgeons.

The shell is typically made of titanium. The metal shell reinforces the polyethylene and prevents any deformity. It can also have a porous surface for bone ingrowth so that cement is not needed to hold it in place. A newer type of cross-linked polyethylene may be more resistant to wear and thus permit the use of larger femoral head sizes.

Research continues into the development of more durable materials and better bearing surfaces for joint replacement components. Alternate bearings such as ceramics and metal on metal will be discussed in questions 49 and 50.

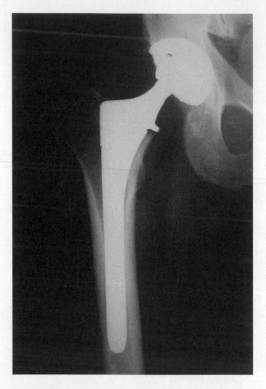

Figure 18   X-ray of a total hip replacement in the body.

© American Academy of Orthopaedic Surgeons.

46. How are the components implanted?

The components of a total hip replacement may be either press fit or cemented into bone. Press fit means that the specific component is impacted tightly into a space of the same size as the component.

At first, all total hip components were cemented in place. The cement acts as a filler or grout, not as a glue. It fills the space between the component and bone.

In early total hip systems, there were only two or three cup sizes and three or four femoral stem sizes available for use. A tight fit was not possible and cement was required to fill the space between component and bone.

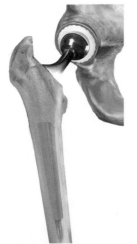

1. Illustration of total hip replacement components.

Courtesy of Smith and Nephew.

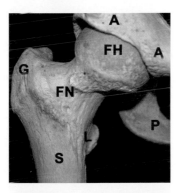

2. Model of a normal hip joint showing: (A) acetabulum or socket, (FH) femoral head, (FN) femoral neck, (G) greater trochanter, (L) lesser trochanter, (P) pelvis, (S) shaft or long portion of femur.

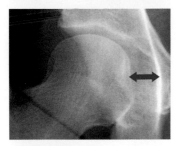

3. X-ray of a normal hip joint. The femoral head is round. Arrows indicate a normal joint space between the head of the femur and the acetabulum.

© American Academy of Orthopaedic Surgeons.

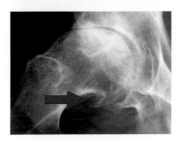

4. X-ray of hip joint with osteoarthritis. The femoral head is no longer round and the joint space is narrow. Arrow points to the large spur at the edge of the femoral head.

5. X-ray of femoral head with avascular necrosis. The joint surface of the femur has collapsed and fractured (red arrow). The fracture line extends into the femoral head (black arrows).

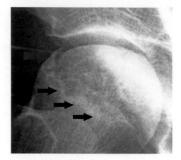

6. DDH. The femoral head and neck are deformed. The socket (red arrows) is long flat and vertical.

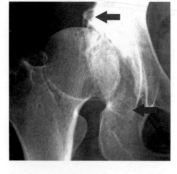

7. X-ray of hip with arthritis secondary to SCFE. The neck of the femur (red arrow) has a round prominent shape.

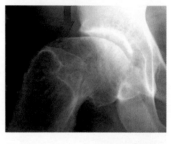

8. X-ray of patient who had previous osteotomy for SCFE. A plate and screws are present in the femur. The proximal femur is severely deformed. Surgery is more difficult because of the need to remove the hardware and the unusual anatomy.

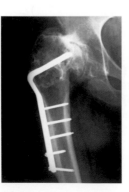

9. The Austin Moore prosthesis was the first partial hip replacement. It was a single or unipolar replacement with no modular parts.

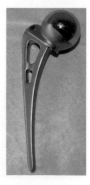

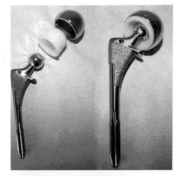

10. A bipolar prosthesis consists of multiple parts (left). The femoral head and stem are below. The white inner bearing fits over the femoral head. The metal shell or outer bearing snaps onto the inner bearing. An assembled bipolar prosthesis is on the right.

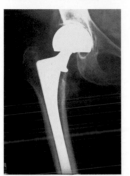

11. X-ray of a bipolar replacement in a hip joint.

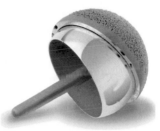

12. Resurfacing components.

Courtesy of Smith and Nephew.

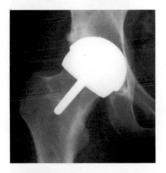

13. X-ray of resurfacing components. The femoral implant covers the femoral head only and preserves bone in the femoral neck.

Courtesy of Smith and Nephew.

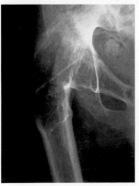

14. X-ray of a hip that has been fused for over fifty years. The femur has been joined to the pelvis to form a single long continuous bone.

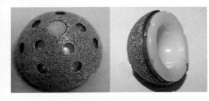

15. Outer titanium metal shell of an acetabular component with a porous surface is seen on the left. Picture at right shows the metal shell with the inner polyethylene liner.

16. A femoral component with a cobalt-chromium head and a titanium stem.

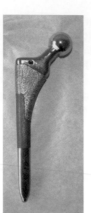

17. Femoral and acetabular components joined together as a total hip arthroplasty.

© *American Academy of Orthopaedic Surgeons.*

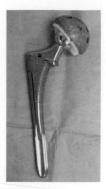

18. X-ray of a total hip replacement in the body.

© *American Academy of Orthopaedic Surgeons.*

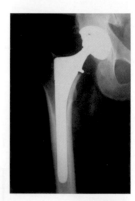

19. Femoral stems have porous surfaces to allow for bone ingrowth into the component. The stem at left is fully coated (F) and has a porous surface on the length of the entire stem. The stem at right is only partially coated (P) between the red arrows.

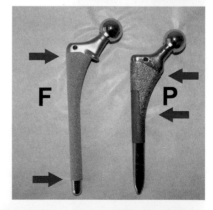

20. Different sized femoral heads ranging from 22–36 mm in diameter.

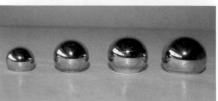

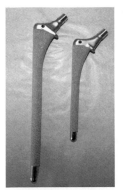

21. Femoral stems in longer and shorter lengths.

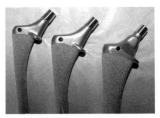

22. Femoral stems in different sizes to match the anatomy of an individual patient.

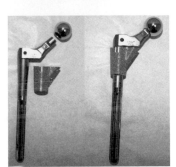

23. A modular prosthesis (S-ROM® Implant) on left consisting of separate head, sleeve, and stem components. The assembled prosthesis is shown at right.

Courtesy of DePuy Orthopaedics, Inc.

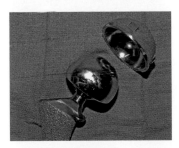

24. A metal femoral head with an all metal acetabular component. Note the large diameter of the femoral head in a metal on metal replacement.

Courtesy of Biomet Orthopedics.

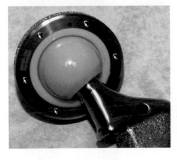

25. Metal femoral component with ceramic head sitting inside metal acetabular component with ceramic liner.

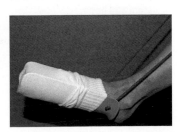

26. An assistive device for putting a sock on the foot without having to bend over.

27. A "grabber" with a trigger handle used to pick up objects from the floor.

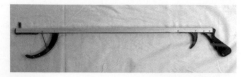

28. Putting on a shoe with a grabber (G) used to steady the shoe in front and a long shoe horn (H) in back.

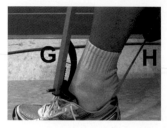

29. X-ray of a total hip dislocation. The ball has come out of the socket.

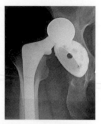

30. Different neck lengths allow the surgeon to adjust leg length and to make the joint more stable.

31. X-ray of a total hip that has developed heterotopic ossification after surgery. A large amount of cloudy white bone (red arrows) is bridging the space between the femur and the acetabulum.

32. A femoral stem in normal position in a femoral canal. A normal cement pattern (red arrows) is seen between the stem and bone.

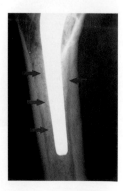

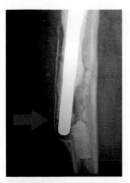

33. A loosened femoral stem. The femur has broken away from the cement and the tip is pushing against the edge of the bone (red arrow). The outer surface of the bone, the cortex, has become very thin.

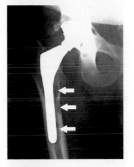

34. Loosening due to thinning of the bone or osteolysis (white arrows).

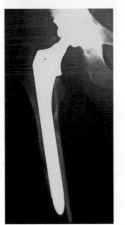

35. Revision of previous case with longer stem prosthesis extending below the defects in the bone.

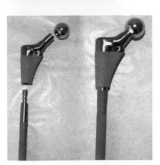

36. A modular revision prosthesis on left (Zimmer ZMR) consisting of separate head, body, and long stem components. The assembled prosthesis is shown at right.

Courtesy of Zimmer Holdings, Inc.

37. An oblong or specially shaped acetabular component can be used to fill a defect in the bone above the acetabulum.

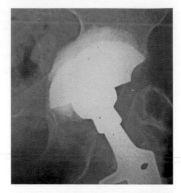

38. A long stem revision component with a cadaver allograft femoral strut (red arrows) on the side. The allograft is fixed with circular cables passed around the bone. It is used to reinforce weakened or osteoporotic bone.

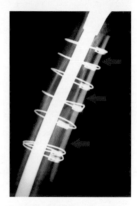

39. Complete fracture across the neck of the femur (red arrow). The head of the femur has broken completely off of the neck and will need replacement.

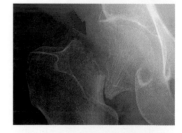

40. Pathologic fracture (red arrow) through abnormal bone in the femoral neck.

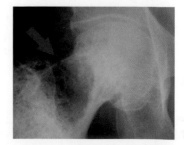

It was noted that over time the interface between cement and bone could break down and the components could become loose. This would cause the need for a revision procedure. Attempts were therefore made to find better fixation for components.

The concept of press fit had been around for a long period of time. Most hemi-arthroplasties done for fractures such as the Austin Moore prosthesis were simply impacted or press fit into bone. It was therefore felt that this might provide better long-term fixation in healthy bone. Noncemented fixation became more popular as implant manufacturers created better instruments and a wider range of component sizes that made a tight press fit possible. Along with this came the development of porous rather than smooth surfaces on the implants. Porous coating allows for ingrowth of bone directly into the implant surface. The optimal pore size for bone ingrowth was determined by laboratory studies.

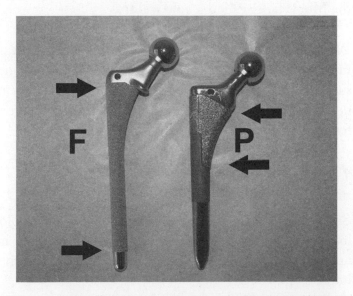

Figure 19 Femoral stems have porous surfaces to allow for bone ingrowth into the component. The stem at left is fully coated (F) and has a porous surface on the length of the entire stem. The stem at right is only partially coated (P) between the arrows.

At present, most acetabular components have porous surfaces along the entire circumference of their interface with bone. Femoral stems may be partially porous coated in some areas or fully coated for the length of the stem.

To insert the acetabular component, the socket is reamed to appropriate size. The metal shell of the acetabular component is then impacted into place. If necessary, an additional one or two screws are placed through holes in the metal shell into the iliac bone of the pelvis to secure fixation. The polyethylene liner of the acetabular component is then placed inside the metal shell and held by a clip or locking mechanism.

In similar fashion, the femoral canal is reamed size for size to accept the stem of the femoral component. The femoral head component is then impacted on to the upper metal portion of the stem called a **Morse taper**. The femoral head forms a metal to metal bond with the Morse taper called a **cold weld**.

While most components at this point in time are press fit, cement remains a useful option in some situations such as soft osteoporotic bone. A total hip that has a noncemented acetabular component and a cemented femoral component is called a *hybrid replacement.*

47. What is bone cement? What is it made from?

Bone cement is an acrylic cement used to hold implants in bone in joint replacement. Bone cement is not really a glue. It is a filler, or grout used to keep the implants in place.

Acrylic cement was originally used for dental work in 1951. Later in the 1960s, Sir John Charnley in

---

Morse taper

Upper metal portion of the femoral stem component where the head and neck are impacted.

Cold weld

The metal to metal bond that is formed when the femoral head component is impacted on the Morse taper part of the femoral stem.

Bone cement is not really a glue. It is a filler, or grout used to keep the implants in place.

Wrightington, England reported the first use of bone cement for joint replacement procedures.

Bone cement is a compound called **polymethyl-methacrylate (PMMA)**. PMMA is a *polymer*. It is a big molecule made up of a long repeating chain of smaller substances called **monomers**. *Monomers* may readily bond to themselves in a process called *polymerization*. Polymers are large molecules and the molecular weight of PMMA is 200,000.

In the operating room, PMMA is prepared by mixing a liquid and a powder. The liquid contains methyl-methacrylate monomer and an activating substance. The powder has smaller particles of PMMA. When the liquid and the monomer are mixed, they form the cement, which is used to implant the components.

The liquid is supplied in a glass vial, the powder in a sealed packet. They are both poured in a mixing bowl to form the cement. The chemical reaction that occurs is an *exothermic* reaction. That means heat is given off as the chemical reaction takes place. The cement is mixed anywhere from one to four minutes. At first it is liquid, then it becomes thick and doughy. A vacuum pump is sometimes attached to the mixing bowl to help remove air bubbles from the cement, which makes the cement stronger.

Early on, cement was placed by finger packing and pressure. Modern techniques have evolved where surgeons now use a special cement gun to inject the cement in the femoral canal. Other techniques allow for pressurizing the cement to make sure that there is a good fill in bone.

If the cement is to be delivered by a cement gun, it is poured as a liquid in to the gun. If the surgeon is going

Polymethyl-methacrylate (PMMA)

Acrylic cement used to hold implants in bone in joint replacement.

Monomer

A small molecule that may bond chemically to other molecules to form a polymer.

to pack the cement by hand, he will mix it longer until it becomes thicker, like modeling clay.

After the cement is placed in the joint, the surgeon will then implant the femoral or acetabular component. He will remove any excess cement.

Bone cement is self-curing. Once the reaction has taken place, the cement begins to set. Usually, it takes between ten and eighteen minutes. Colder temperatures slow the reaction down, while warmer temperatures make the cement set faster. The surgeon will maintain pressure on the implanted component until the cement is dry.

PMMA is biologically compatible. Allergic reactions or sensitivity to the cement are rare. Operating room nurses have sometimes complained of headaches from cement fumes given off after the liquid and powder are mixed. Despite this, there is no evidence that the fumes have any toxicity.

In rare instances, implantation of the cement has been known to cause a sudden drop in blood pressure. The reason is not well known. The anesthesiologist will take steps to make sure that the patient is well-hydrated and blood pressure maintained while the cement is being implanted.

Attempts have been made to improve the fixation of the cement to the surface of the femoral component. Femoral stems were coated with a layer of acrylic during the manufacturing process. It was felt that the cement would bond to a like substance on the surface of the metal better than it would bond to the metal itself. Long-term results however were mixed.

A radiopaque material such as barium sulfate is included with the powder used to make the cement. This is done so that the cement will be visible on x-ray and any changes in the cement mantle can be identified later on.

Antibiotics can be mixed with the cement in cases where there is an infection. The two most common antibiotics used in cement are Gentamycin and Tobramycin. The antibiotics will gradually extrude from cement into the soft tissues over time. Antibiotic laden cement is used as a spacer in infection cases. If the joint replacement has become infected, it is sometimes necessary to remove all of the components and wait several weeks before they can be reimplanted. The antibiotic spacers are shaped and inserted in the joint to temporarily fill the empty space when the components are taken out.

When bone cement was first developed for use with orthopaedic implants, FDA approval was required for its use. Ironically, as noncemented components with porous surfaces were developed, FDA approval was required to implant components that did not require cement.

Bone cement has other uses in orthopaedic surgery besides joint replacement. It has sometimes been used to fill defects in bone in fracture cases. Recently, a new procedure, **kyphoplasty**, has been used to treat compression fractures in the spine. In this procedure, bone cement is injected directly in to the vertebral body to restore the normal height of the vertebra that has collapsed from the fracture.

Kyphoplasty
A procedure to treat compression fractures in the spine where bone cement is injected into the vertebral body.

48. Why are components modular?

Modular parts are interchangeable pieces that go together to make up one structure. Both the femoral and the acetabular components of a total hip arthroplasty may be modular.

The Operation

The original total hip components were *monoblock*. Each component was one single piece and a surgeon had relatively few choices. The addition of modularity gives the surgeon more options and allows him to best match the components to the patient's individual anatomy. A surgeon may use modular components to help him solve specific problems such as leg length discrepancy or an unusual angle (version) of the femur. Modular components can be used to provide a better fit and to create greater stability in the hip replacement.

The addition of modularity gives the surgeon more options and allows him to best match the components to the patient's individual anatomy.

The option of modularity gives the surgeon greater flexibility. He can fine tune the arthroplasty or replacement to meet the specific needs of the patient. Some of the features that can be addressed by modularity are:

- Size of the femoral head (affects both the head and the acetabular liner)
- Length of the femoral neck
- Offset of the femoral neck
- Width of the proximal or metaphyseal part of the femoral component
- Fit of the femoral stem
- Length of the femoral stem
- Shape of the femoral stem—straight or bowed
- Shape of the liner of the socket—elevated rim or lateralized
- Angle or the version of the femoral neck

Most acetabular components have two modular parts, the outer metal shell and the inner polyethylene liner. Femoral components also have two parts, the femoral head and the stem of the component. Some femoral components, which are mostly used for revision cases, have three modular parts. In these components, the middle section below the head, called the body or

The Operation

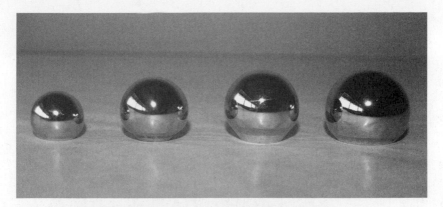

Figure 20   Different sized femoral heads ranging from 22–36 mm in diameter.

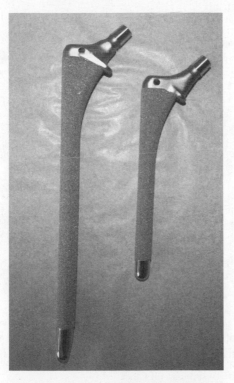

Figure 21   Femoral stems in longer and shorter lengths.

metaphysis, is separate from the femoral stem. The middle component comes in several shapes and sizes that can be used to make up for bone loss or bone height in a revision case.

117

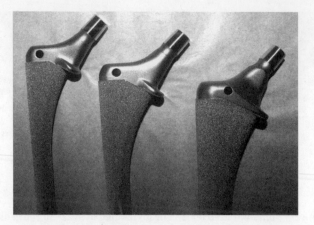

Figure 22   Femoral stems in different sizes to match the anatomy of an individual patient.

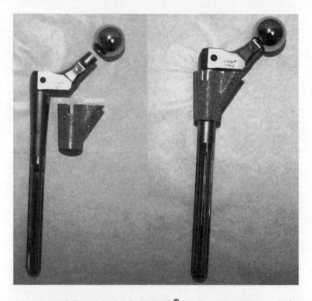

Figure 23   A modular prosthesis (S-ROM® Implant) on left consisting of separate head, sleeve, and stem components. The assembled prosthesis is shown at right.

Courtesy of DePuy Orthopaedics, Inc.

Three piece modular femoral components can be a handy tool for a surgeon in a situation where bone loss makes it hard to fit normal components. The weakest points of these components are the junctions between the modular parts.

Modularity means that most setups for a routine total hip replacement may have over one thousand possible combinations of head, neck, acetabular, and femoral stem sizes. The surgeon can make the best possible choices for fit and fixation of all components.

49. Can a hip replacement be metal on metal?

Metal on metal total hip replacements have been in use for approximately 50 years. Because the combination of metal on polyethylene has been so effective and so popular, far fewer metal on metal total hip replacements have been performed.

The two opposing sides of a total hip replacement are called the *bearing surfaces*. The goal of a total hip arthroplasty is to create bearing surfaces which have low friction, good lubrication, will not break down, and will last a long time. The bearing surfaces must be

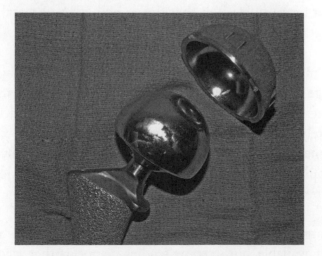

Figure 24   A metal femoral head with an all metal acetabular component. Note the large diameter of the femoral head in a metal on metal replacement.

Courtesy of Biomet Orthopedics.

compatible and must not give off particles when they wear that would cause problems within the joint or other parts of the body.

A metal femoral head articulating with ultra high molecular weight polyethylene has become the modern standard for total hip arthroplasty. As the polyethylene wears, however, it gives off small particles called **particulate debris**. The debris remains in the area around the joint. It causes thinning of the bone or **osteolysis**. When osteolysis occurs in either the femur or the acetabulum, it can cause loosening of the components and ultimately result in the need for revision surgery.

Alternative combinations of bearing surfaces are being studied in an effort to eliminate wear debris and the thinning of the bone that it causes.

A metal on metal prosthesis made of cobalt-chromium alloy was first developed by McKee and Farrar in the early 1960s. Since that time, newer designs have been put forward. It is felt that the combination of metal on metal will result in less wear debris.

A metal on metal hip joint replacement has the advantage of using larger sizes for the femoral head. Larger sizes mean that the hip joint is more stable and less likely to come out of the socket or dislocate. A second benefit is that the edge of the socket is less likely to impinge on the head or neck of the femur as the joint moves into extreme positions.

Large series of cases with long-term follow up are not yet available, but in some studies it appears that second generation metal on metal replacements will last as long as metal on polyethylene.

Particulate debris

Small particles given off in the area of the joint when the polyethylene liner of an acetabular component wears down. It is felt to cause thinning of bone and loosening of components.

Osteolysis

Thinning or loss of bone usually caused by infection or particulate debris.

A metal on metal hip joint replacement has the advantage of using larger sizes for the femoral head. Larger sizes mean that the hip joint is more stable and less likely to come out of the socket or dislocate.

Metal surfaces, like polyethylene, can give off small particles of debris. The tiny metal particles are called *ions*. While they do not cause a reaction in the joint such as osteolysis or loosening, some particles may appear in other parts of the body. Metallic ions have been found in blood serum, in red blood cells and in urine. It is not known if their presence will have toxicity or effect on any organs. Beyond this, it is not known if metal particles accumulating in the body would have a cancer causing or carcinogenic effect.

In a few rare cases, the metal may cause a local hypersensitivity reaction.

Metal on metal bearings have recently become more popular because they are used in hip resurfacing procedures. As noted above, the long-term effects of metal on metal in the human body are not known.

More information is needed on the *tribology* or the friction, lubrication, and wear of metal on metal surfaces.

50. What are ceramics?

Ceramics are hard materials that are inorganic and nonmetallic. They are materials which are formed by the action of heat. The word ceramic comes from the Greek *keramikos*. Examples of ceramics are clay, glass, cement, and porcelain. Ceramics are used in many structures including bricks, tiles, china dishes, and pottery. Ceramic materials can also be used for medical and scientific purposes.

Ceramics have a high resistance to wear and corrosion.

Ceramics have a high resistance to wear and corrosion. They tend to be more heat resistant than most metals. They are, however, very hard and brittle.

Ceramic on ceramic arthroplasties are another attempt to use alternative bearing surfaces to reduce wear and debris. Ceramics have been used for more than 30 years, but recent designs have become more popular. Both ceramic on ceramic and ceramic on polyethylene combinations have been tried.

The two most common types of ceramic that are used in hip replacements are *alumina* and *zirconia*. These materials are hard and inert. They have good wettability and the opposing surfaces are well lubricated against one another. They are resistant to wear and to corrosion and are not known to cause any local reaction. In contrast to metal, there is no ion release which could cause long-term effects in other organs of the body.

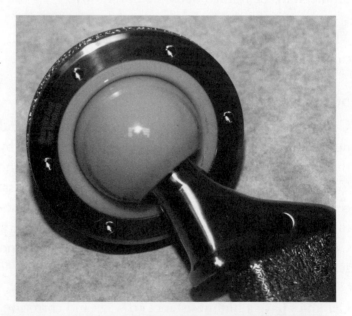

Figure 25 **Metal femoral component with ceramic head sitting inside metal acetabular component with ceramic liner.**

Although ceramic materials are very hard and firm, they are also very brittle. There has been a small incidence of component fracture when ceramics are used. In addition, ceramic on ceramic bearings are sometimes noted to have a clicking or squeaking effect. This occurs in a small number of ceramic replacements. The cause is not clear.

It is felt that careful placement of the components to avoid scratching and impingement will help prevent a ceramic hip from squeaking.

Further research and long-term studies are required to determine the relative risks and benefits of alternative bearings such as ceramics and metal on metal. The goal is to provide bearing surfaces that will be durable and not have any long-term local or systemic effects.

PART EIGHT

After Surgery

What kind of medication will I be given for pain?

What precautions do I need to take against dislocation?

What kind of physical therapy will I need?

More . . .

51. How long will I need to be in the hospital?

Most patients who undergo total hip arthroplasty will need to be in the hospital for 3 to 4 days following surgery. After their hospital stay, many patients choose to go to a secondary rehabilitation facility for physical therapy and gait training. Most patients stay at the rehabilitation facility until they are strong enough to function at home.

Other patients choose to go directly home from the hospital. Arrangements are then made at home for wound care, physical therapy, and administration of blood thinners.

In some settings, patients may choose to go home 1 to 2 days after total hip replacement. This decision is based on how strong they feel, the progress of their rehabilitation, and how much help is available at home.

In general, older patients with multiple medical problems tend to require a longer time in the hospital than younger patients who are in good general health.

Linda C., a patient, says:

I spent three days in the hospital, a week at inpatient rehabilitation, and six weeks in outpatient physical therapy. After two weeks, I was walking without a cane. At two months, I was deemed recovered! I could do steps in my office building, the elliptical machine, and long walks on a regular basis. By the third month, I was back mowing the lawn and gardening, and I could walk a mile without feeling fatigue in the hip.

52. What kind of medication will I be given for pain?

Pain medication after hip replacement surgery can be given through an epidural catheter, through an intravenous line (IV), or by mouth.

Postoperative pain is greatest in the first 2 or 3 days after surgery. If you have had epidural anesthesia during surgery, the epidural catheter may be left in place for an additional 24–48 hours. Either a local anesthetic, morphine or both can be given through the catheter. This provides good pain relief in the immediate postoperative period.

If you have had general anesthesia, then you will most likely require some form of IV medication as you start your recovery. An IV line is left in place and the medication can be given through the line so that you do not require multiple needle sticks. IV medication is stronger than oral medication and provides greater pain relief. It may be given as single doses by your nurse as needed.

A common way to give IV pain medication is *patient controlled analgesia* (PCA), which allows you to give yourself pain medication as you need it.

A PCA line has a small computer that is part of the intravenous pump. The PCA dose is ordered by the surgeon and the machine is set by the nurse. The computer pump controls the medication dose, the time interval between doses, and the maximum hourly dose of medication that can be given. It can also supply a dose of pain medication at a constant rate.

You are given a button at your bedside and press the button when you need pain medication. PCA is safe because the computer will not allow you to overdose. Still it is important that only you and not your family or friends press the PCA button so that you do not get more medication than you need.

The pain medications usually given through a PCA pump are morphine and hydromorphone (Dilaudid).

After 2 or 3 days, the pain will be a lot better. You will be able to switch from IV to oral or P.O. pain medication. P.O. comes from the Latin term *per os* meaning *by mouth*. You will no longer need the IV line and can start taking pills. Common pain medications given by mouth are Percocet, Dilaudid, Vicodin, and Tylenol No. 3 with Codeine. Side effects from these medications can be fatigue, nausea, or constipation. There can also be allergy or sensitivity.

NSAIDs can be used along with these medications to relieve pain and inflammation after surgery.

As your recovery progresses, you will need less pain medication. You may only need to take a pill after prolonged activity or when you go to sleep. It is sometimes good to take pain medication before the start of a physical therapy session so that you feel better when you are doing your exercises.

Try to limit prescription pain medication as soon as you can. Any of these drugs can become a habit or even an addiction.

Try to limit prescription pain medication as soon as you can. Any of these drugs can become a habit or even an addiction. You can take over-the-counter medication such as aspirin, Tylenol, or ibuprofen if you have any residual pain.

53. When will I get out of bed?

Most total hip replacement patients get out of bed on the day of surgery or the first day after. It is felt that faster mobilization speeds rehabilitation and prevents medical complications.

You will first get out of bed with assistance and move to a chair. You will then stand with a walker or crutches. Some surgeons will allow you to put full weight on your operated leg right away. Other times, you will be partial weight bearing and increase weight as your surgeon allows.

You will have physical therapy for gait training and instruction in how to walk with a walker or crutches.

If you have had an extensive reconstruction, your surgeon may delay any weight bearing at all until your hip is healed and it is safe to bear weight.

Getting out of bed helps to prevent medical complications, such as fever, pneumonia, pressure sores, and blood clots. The more you walk and move about, the less likely you are to form a clot in your legs.

Sometimes, getting out of bed is delayed by the presence of a surgical drain or excessive pain or swelling in your hip. If this happens, you will be encouraged to take deep breaths to prevent problems with your lungs and to turn in bed to protect the skin from pressure areas.

Getting out of bed is the first and most important step towards your rehabilitation.

Linda W., a patient, says:

It was a bit scary, but after the first couple of steps your mind really does believe that the replacement is going to support you. I also remember that the hip pain was gone—the pain at the incision was nothing compared to the hip pain.

Boris K., a patient, says:

It did feel different at the first time—loose and weak. It was not the artificial hip itself, but the tissues surrounding and supporting it.

54. Why do I need antibiotics? How long will they last?

Antibiotics are routinely given before total hip arthroplasty to help prevent infection. Infection is a serious and potentially devastating complication. Most studies have shown that giving antibiotics immediately before and for a period of time just after surgery can substantially reduce the risk of infection.

Antibiotics that are given to protect you from infection are called **prophylactic antibiotics**.

Prophylactic antibiotics

Antibiotics given before and after surgery to protect against infection.

Cefazolin (Ancef) is the most commonly given antibiotic for patients undergoing total hip arthroplasty. It is similar to penicillin, but has a broader spectrum of coverage. It cannot, however, be given to patients with a confirmed allergy to penicillin.

In this instance, Vancomycin or Clindamycin can be used as substitutes. Prophylactic antibiotics are given intravenously within one hour before the skin incision is made. They are continued for a period of up to 24 hours after surgery. There is no evidence that taking antibiotics for longer than 24 hours reduces the risk of infection. It may, in fact, contribute to the growth of resistant organisms within the body.

Antibiotics would only be restarted if you were to develop an infection in the postoperative period.

Antibiotic prophylaxis given at the proper time has been shown to reduce the overall instance of infection in hip replacement surgery.

55. Will I need a blood transfusion?

Approximately 50% of the people undergoing total hip arthroplasty will need a blood transfusion either during or after surgery.

Several factors can affect the need for transfusion. If you are starting with a low blood count, or *hematocrit*, then you are more likely to need blood after surgery. The amount of blood loss during surgery can be variable. It may simply depend on how much the bone and soft tissues around your hip bleed during your operation. While most blood loss occurs during surgery, additional blood is lost in the soft tissues underneath the skin in the period after surgery.

Your surgeon may place a reinfusion drain in your hip at the end of the procedure. This will allow any blood that has been drained to be returned to you in the first few hours after surgery.

Your blood count will be checked for the first 3 or 4 days after surgery. This will determine whether or not a transfusion is necessary.

Younger patients who are in good general health may often tolerate a lower blood count than older patients or patients with multiple medical problems. It is important to have enough blood to bring oxygen to vital organs such as your heart and brain.

A higher blood count will bring a greater oxygen carrying capacity to these vital organs. It will also give you more strength as you proceed with your rehabilitation.

Many patients choose to undergo autologous blood donation in the period before surgery. They give one or two units of their own blood to a blood bank, so it will be available for transfusion during surgery and in the postoperative period.

Your family or friends may also choose to give blood for *directed* blood transfusion. This means that the blood they give will be reserved specifically for you. It does depend of course on blood testing and compatibility.

Interestingly enough, most studies show little difference in the incidence of transmitted disease between blood from anonymous donors to the blood bank and directed donors.

56. Will I need a catheter?

A catheter is a tube inserted in your bladder to drain urine if you are unable to void after surgery. It may be needed for a short time.

Most patients don't need a catheter but some have difficulty passing urine or voiding in the postoperative period. When this occurs, a catheter can be useful.

It may be difficult to void when you are lying down right after surgery. Anesthesia or pain medication may affect the muscles that help you void. Urine builds up in your bladder. This is called *retention*. It creates a sensation of pressure which may be very uncomfortable.

A catheter is sometimes helpful for patients who are incontinent or have to void repeatedly.

Older men who have enlarged prostate glands may have difficulty voiding after surgery. A catheter is sometimes helpful for patients who are incontinent or have to void repeatedly. After surgery it is difficult for them to get up to go to the bathroom.

When urine builds up in the bladder, the bladder becomes enlarged or *distended*. Sometimes the swelling or distention of the bladder can be felt in the lower abdomen. A noninvasive ultrasound test called a *bladder scan* can determine how much urine is in the bladder and if a catheter is needed.

The catheter may be placed once and then removed. This is called *straight catheterization*. Other times the catheter may be left in place. The catheter is usually kept for 1 or 2 days after surgery. Most patients are not discharged from the hospital until they can void without the catheter.

If you cannot void without the catheter, it is necessary to consult a urinary specialist called a *urologist*.

57. What kind of blood thinners will I have to take? How long will I have to take them?

Several types of blood thinners are available to help protect against **deep vein thrombosis (DVT)** or blood clots forming in the legs. Some of the medications can be taken by mouth. Others are given by needle injections under the skin called subcutaneous injections.

Deep vein thrombosis (DVT)

When blood clots form in the deep veins of the leg.

While most surgeons agree that prophylaxis for DVT should be given for a short period of time after surgery, the evidence is not clear as to how long a period of time the medication should continue.

Blood thinners are often combined with compression stockings or pneumatic compression devices that intermittently squeeze the legs. These devices are called **mechanical prophylaxis** because they are not drugs. They prevent blood from becoming static and forming clots.

Mechanical prophylaxis

Mechanical devices such as compression boots used to prevent blood clots.

Most surgeons agree that blood thinners combined with early mobilization and some mechanical prophylaxis offer the best protection.

Warfarin or *Coumadin* is used by many orthopaedic surgeons in the postoperative period. Coumadin has the benefit that it can be given orally. Most surgeons start Coumadin on the day after surgery. A loading dose of approximately 5 to 10 mg is given. It may take 2 to 3 days to reach a therapeutic level. Doses are monitored and adjusted on a daily basis.

The test used to monitor and adjust the dose of Coumadin is called the International Normalized Ratio or *INR* for short. A blood sample is taken each day and the INR is checked to make sure that it is at the right level. The daily dose is then prescribed by the surgeon. If the INR is high, a lower dose will be given. Conversely, if the INR is not yet in therapeutic range, the surgeon will prescribe a higher dose.

Coumadin works by inhibiting vitamin K and its action on the clotting system. Its effects can partially be overcome by giving vitamin K. The main side effect or complication from Coumadin can be uncontrolled bleeding if levels are too high. Coumadin has been shown to be effective in preventing DVT and is used by approximately 50% of orthopaedic surgeons following hip surgery.

In recent years, low molecular weight heparin has become popular for postoperative DVT prophylaxis. It is more stable and lasts longer than regular heparin. Despite this, its half life, or the time at which only 50% remains in the bloodstream, is approximately four and a half hours.

Low molecular weight heparin is available in two compounds, enoxaparin (Lovenox) and dalteparin (Fragmin). It works by inhibiting clotting factors Xa and 2a.

Unlike Coumadin, low molecular weight heparin is given on a once or twice-daily basis by subcutaneous injection. Its effect on blood clotting cannot be monitored by tests such as the INR. Accordingly, a standard dose is given. This is usually 30 mg twice a day for Lovenox and 5000 International Units once a day for Fragmin.

The main side effect or complication of low molecular weight heparin is low platelets or **thrombocytopenia**. It is necessary to monitor the platelet count while these drugs are being given. If there is excessive bleeding, the effects of low molecular weight heparin can be partially reversed by giving protamine sulfate.

Fondaparinux (Arixtra) is another drug that is given subcutaneously. It is classified as a synthetic pentasaccharide that works by inhibiting factor Xa. Like low molecular weight heparin, it is given by subcutaneous injection. The standard dose is 2.5 mg once a day. As with low molecular weight heparin, the principal side effect can be excessive bleeding.

Aspirin is another drug used by many orthopaedic surgeons as a blood thinner.

Aspirin, like Coumadin, can be given orally. It works by inhibiting platelet aggregation. That is it helps prevent platelets in the blood stream from coming together to form clots. It is typically given in a dose of 325 mg twice a day and has been shown in some studies to be an effective chemical prophylaxis. As with low

Thrombocytopenia
A condition where there is a low platelet count in blood.

Aspirin is another drug used by many orthopaedic surgeons as a blood thinner.

molecular weight heparin, the effects of aspirin in the blood stream cannot be monitored. The main side effect is gastric upset. Aspirin should not be given to patients with history of ulcer disease, colitis, or other gastrointestinal problems.

The timing, dosage, and choice of drug for DVT prophylaxis following hip surgery remain controversial. The American Academy of Orthopaedic Surgeons issued clinical guidelines in 2007 on "Prevention of Symptomatic Pulmonary Embolism in Patients Undergoing Total Hip or Knee Arthroplasty." This was an effort to clarify which treatments are effective in preventing DVT and reducing the incidence of pulmonary embolism. Pulmonary embolism which can be fatal is the most serious consequence of DVT.

The AAOS guidelines suggest different treatment regimens based on a patient's individual risk for pulmonary embolism and for major bleeding.

They recommend that prophylaxis be started 12 to 24 hours after the conclusion of surgery. This may be delayed if there is an epidural catheter in place near the spine. In this case, prophylaxis should not be started until several hours after the catheter has been removed.

Recommended drugs are aspirin, Coumadin, low molecular weight heparin (Lovenox, Fragmin), and pentasaccharides (Arixtra). It is recommended that all of these drugs be given for an initial period of at least 7 to 12 days and possibly as long as 6 weeks.

Inferior vena cava

A large vein that carries blood from the lower part of the body to the right side of the heart.

The Academy also recommends that patients who are unable to tolerate anticoagulation be considered for placement of an **inferior vena cava** *filter*.

A filter, or umbrella, is a metallic surgical device placed in the largest vein of the lower part of the body, the inferior vena cava. The umbrella allows blood to pass through but blocks the passage of a clot large enough to affect the lung. It is introduced through a small incision in the groin and then placed at appropriate level by the surgeon.

While anticoagulation has been shown to be beneficial in hip replacement patients, the best duration of therapy remains unclear. Most studies show a benefit in the first 7 to 12 days after surgery, but the optimal length of treatment has not yet been determined.

The American College of Chest Physicians recommends prophylaxis for 7 to 10 days after surgery but 28 to 35 days in patients who are at higher risk.

Your orthopaedic surgeon can provide information on the type of drug and duration of therapy you will need after surgery.

58. Will I need to use a walker or crutches?

Everyone who has had hip surgery needs an assistive aid such as a walker or crutches in the period right after surgery.

For the first few days, you will have pain in your hip and weakness in the muscles of your thigh. You will need support to stand, balance, and bear weight. You will also need support as you take steps and begin to walk.

In the hospital a physical therapist will start you off with a walker or crutches. He or she will tell you how to use the assistive devices and how to be safe. Sometimes your surgeon will recommend that you be nonweight bearing or partial weight bearing for a period of time. This will mean that you need the walker or crutches a little longer. If, for example, the bone in your hip is deficient and a bone graft has to be placed, weight bearing will need to be protected until the graft has had a chance to heal and the bone becomes strong.

If full weight bearing is permitted, you may advance to a cane as soon as you are comfortable and your surgeon thinks you are ready. Most people require crutches or a walker for at least 2 to 3 weeks, but younger patients frequently advance to a cane after a shorter period of time. You will be most comfortable using a cane in the hand opposite the side of your operation. That is, if you have had right hip surgery you will want to use the cane on your left side. Try it both ways, but you will always find that you feel more comfortable and your walking is better with a cane in the opposite hand.

Some patients start out with a four prong or quad cane because it is more stable than a straight cane. As your balance improves, however, a straight cane may be more comfortable.

You may try walking without the cane. At first, your gait may show a lurch. Your body tips to the operated side as you walk. This is due to the mechanics of the hip and the weakened muscles around the incision. Almost always the lurch is relieved when you use a cane. As you get stronger, the lurch will lessen and may only be evident when you get tired at the end of the day.

Your surgeon will advise you when it is safe to go from crutches to a cane or when it is safe to use nothing at all.

Your surgeon will advise you when it is safe to go from crutches to a cane or when it is safe to use nothing at all. In some cases he may rely on input from the physical therapist who has been working with you.

59. What precautions do I need to take against dislocation?

While you are in the hospital your surgeon and your therapist will outline some of the precautions you need to take to protect your new hip. First and foremost, you need to take precautions to prevent dislocation.

Dislocation means that the ball of the hip comes out of the socket. During surgery, the capsule, which holds the normal hip joint in place, is divided. For 3 months after surgery, until the capsule heals, you have to make sure that you do not do anything that would cause your new hip to dislocate.

Any extreme movement or position could result in a dislocation.

There are several rules you should follow:

- Do not bend your hip more than 90 degrees.
- Do not sit in low chairs.
- Sit in higher chairs or use cushions to raise the level of your seat.
- Do not sit with your knees above the level of your hips.
- Do not cross your legs.
- Do not bring your operated leg across the midline of your body.
- Do not kneel.
- Sleep with pillows between your knees.
- Use assistive aids such as a grabber or long shoe horn.
- Avoid twisting motions when you are standing or walking.
- Do not turn your leg inward when you are walking.
- When you are turning in a seated position, turn your entire body not just your operative leg.

- Extend your leg when you are sitting, when you are getting up, or when you are going to sit down.
- Keep objects in your house especially in your kitchen at a level where you do not have to bend over to get them.

Most surgeons recommend that patients take dislocation precautions for 3 months, but after you have had a total hip replacement, it is a good idea not to cross your leg or bend your hip more than 90 degrees at any time.

Obviously, a fall or any significant trauma can also cause a dislocation or injure other parts of your body. While you are recovering, your strength and balance will take time to get back to normal, and it is a good idea to take a few measures to prevent an unwanted fall.

You may want to arrange the furniture in your house so that it will not be in your way while you are walking. You should make sure there are no loose rugs on the surface of the floor. Be extra careful when you are walking on any slippery surface. Make sure there are no loose cords or wires in an exposed area of any room. It helps to install hand rails on any staircase in your house and on steps leading up to your house. Remind your family to be careful not to leave any loose objects such as toys or shoes on the floor.

Of course you may need to restrain any pets. Even though you love your dog, he can cause you to lose your balance if he jumps on you or jumps in your way.

At night, keep a small night light on in your bedroom and hallways. You should also use assistive walking aids such as a cane or walker if you are getting up at night. Never mix alcohol and pain medication!

In the first few days after surgery, keep the wound clean and dry to help prevent infection. Leave a dressing over the wound until your doctor tells you it is safe to remove it. Do not get the wound area wet or apply any ointment to the wound without permission from your surgeon. Also do not wear tight clothing that might irritate or abrade the wound. Avoid fabrics to which you might be sensitive and which might cause a rash around the wound.

Remember too that any kind of trauma to the wound area, even minor, can cause the wound to open up and lead to infection or the need for more surgery.

60. Can I go home from the hospital or should I go to a rehabilitation facility?

Thirty years ago, it was common to stay 2 weeks in the hospital after total hip replacement. You would stay in the acute care hospital until you were able to walk, your wound had healed, and the stitches or staples used to close the wound were removed. Things have changed a lot since then.

Most patients now have less need for a prolonged stay in an acute care hospital. They stay only 3 or 4 days unless they have other medical problems. Many younger patients on aggressive rehabilitation schedules stay only 1 or 2 days in the hospital before they go home.

Many total hip patients can go directly home after a short hospitalization. Others need more time to recover. The purpose of going to a rehabilitation facility is to gain strength and to improve your overall level of function before you go home.

The purpose of going to a rehabilitation facility is to gain strength and to improve your overall level of function before you go home.

At the rehabilitation facility, your care will be supervised by a specialist in rehabilitation medicine called a *physiatrist*. A specialist in internal medicine, an internist, may also participate in your care if you have any medical problems. At the rehab facility, physical therapy is intensive and may take several hours a day. You will be discharged when you can walk independently and do basic activities such as bathing, dressing, and going up and down stairs.

If you go straight home from the hospital instead of to a rehab facility you will need:

- Pain medication.
- Anticoagulation—you will either need to take oral medication such as Coumadin or aspirin or be given injections such as Lovenox.
- Home physical therapy—a therapist will come to your home to teach you walking and strengthening exercises.
- Assistive devices such as a reacher or grabber, sock donner, and long shoe horn.
- Help with basic activities like bathing, dressing, and preparing meals.

The most important factor in whether you go home or to rehabilitation facility is how well you do in physical therapy. If you can walk independently, it will be much easier for you to go straight home. Your physical strength and stamina play a role in this regard. You should also take into consideration your home situation. If you live alone and have no one to help you or if you have to climb two flights of stairs to reach your bedroom it may be better to spend some time at a rehab facility and become more independent.

Lastly, your insurance coverage will be a factor. Some insurance carriers will only cover a limited stay at a secondary facility or will insist that you go to a subacute rather than an acute rehabilitation setting.

A social worker or case manager will meet with you during your hospitalization. He or she can review your progress and assess your needs and can help you decide which option, home or rehab, will give you the fastest and safest recovery.

61. What kind of physical therapy will I need?

Physical therapy starts right after surgery while you are in the hospital. Therapy will continue if you go to a rehabilitation facility and later in your home. When you are strong enough, you can go to an outpatient physical therapy facility. Therapy consists of learning how to walk, exercises to strengthen your new hip and instructions in activities and precautions. Needless to add, it is necessary to make a strong effort at physical therapy in order to achieve a good result from your surgery.

When you first start therapy, you will be shown exercises for your hip that you can do in bed. You will be shown how to safely sit up in bed and how to safely get out of bed and to stand.

You will also begin to walk on the day of surgery or on the first day after. Your therapist will start you out with a walker or crutches. Your therapy will depend on how much weight you are allowed to put on your leg (nonweight, partial, or full).

Your therapist will show you how to get in and out of a chair without bending your hip too much. He will show you how to go up and down stairs. This is important if you live in a two-level house. He will also show you how to get in and out of a car.

Either your physical therapist or an occupational therapist will help you with activities of daily living (ADL). These include dressing, bathing, and performing routine household chores. To do these things you will be shown how to use a variety of assistive devices.

Your therapist will explain hip precautions or the things you have to do to prevent a dislocation of your hip.

Your therapist will also show you exercises that you can do on your own.

62. What exercises should I do to strengthen my hip?

Exercise is key to your recovery. You may only have 2 or 3 hours of supervised therapy a week. It is important to exercise on your own several times a day. Try to put aside a few minutes every 2 or 3 hours. Become familiar with the exercises and set up a routine. You'll find the time goes quickly!

The following is a list of standard total hip strengthening exercises:

Exercises in Bed

These exercises should be done lying on your back in bed or on a flat surface.

- Heel slides—slide your heel back and forth on the bed
- Ankle pumps—flex your ankle up and down
- Gluteal sets—contract your buttock and hip muscles
- Straight leg raises—lift your leg off the bed with your knee fully straightened

- Abduction slides—slide your leg sideways on the bed away from your body

Exercises Sitting

Sit upright in a chair with your knee at a right angle. Remember not to flex your knee above the level of your hip.

- Short arc knee extensions—start with your knee at a right angle and fully straighten your leg
- Full arc knee extensions—start with your knee fully flexed and straighten your leg

Exercises Standing

Do these exercises standing while you are holding on to a counter or the back of a chair.

- Knee raises—with your hip straight flex your knee
- Hip abduction—lift your leg sideways away from your body
- Hip extension—lift your leg behind your body

63. What kind of assistive aids will I need?

There are many assistive aids that can help you in your recovery from total hip arthroplasty. Since you want to be careful not to bend your hip too much, several instruments are available to help you do things that you would otherwise be unable to do. Some of these include:

- Leg lifter—a tool that looks like a leash or stick with a loop at the end. The loop grabs your foot so that you can pull your leg up on a bed or onto a flat surface. A leg lifter is useful when you do not have full strength of your hip flexors so you cannot yet raise your leg.
- Sock donner—an instrument with a ring frame at the end which allows you to slide a sock onto your foot without bending over.

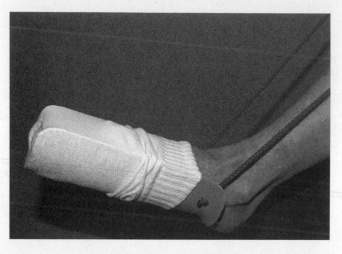

Figure 26 An assistive device for putting a sock on the foot without having to bend over.

- Long shoe horn—to help you squeeze into your shoe without having to bend over to stretch the back of the shoe. Many patients who have a bad hip use a long shoe horn before surgery.
- Long handle sponge—a shower sponge at the end of a long handle to help with bathing.
- Scratcher—like a back scratcher to help you scratch without turning or bending.
- Reacher or grabber—a long metal device with a trigger handle at one end and a grasping mechanism at the other. This helps you pick up objects from the floor without having to bend over.

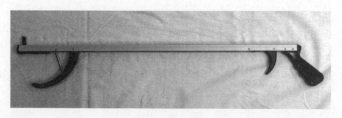

Figure 27 A "grabber" with a trigger handle used to pick up objects from the floor.

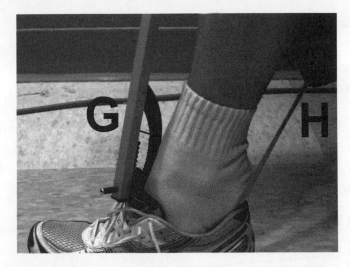

Figure 28 **Putting on a shoe with a grabber (G) used to steady the shoe in front and a long shoe horn (H) in back.**

- Shower chair—a plastic chair that allows you to sit in the shower while you are bathing.
- Bath bench—like a chair that fits over the side of your bathtub. A bench rests on the edge of the tub. It allows you to sit and then swing over to the edge for bathing.
- Raised toilet seat—so you do not have to bend as much while you are sitting.
- Commode—when you first get home, a bedside commode may be useful so you do not have to walk to the bathroom.

It is helpful to know how to use each of these tools before you leave the hospital or rehabilitation facility. A physical or occupational therapist can give you instruction and show you what to do.

Arrange to have these assistive aids waiting for you before you get home because you will need them right away.

64. When can I go back to work?

You can return to work after hip surgery as soon as you are comfortable. It really depends on where you work and what type of work you do.

Obviously you can return to office work faster than you can do physical work or manual labor. It also takes longer to return to a job that requires hours of standing.

Many people with computer access begin working from home less than a week after surgery.

Many people with computer access begin working from home less than a week after surgery. It all depends on how good you feel and how much energy you have. Most people, however, cannot work from home and must wait until they are ready to return to their office or place of work.

Getting there may be part of the problem. For the first 4 weeks or so, you will be unable to drive and will have to arrange for someone to take you to work. The physical setup of your job may be a barrier. If you have to go up and down several flights of stairs every day or if you have to walk across a long or icy parking lot, it may take time before you can get back to your job.

In the first few weeks after surgery, you may get tired easily. You may find that your stamina is not as great as you would like it to be. You may only want to go back to work on a limited basis or work part time.

Talk to your employer about arranging your schedule. He or she may allow you to come in later when getting to work might be easier. It may be possible to manage your schedule so that you can get most of your work done but still have a shorter day. He may arrange your job so that you have to do less standing or walking until you are fully recovered. It may also be possible to do less traveling if you work outside of the office.

Returning to work and your regular routine is a normal part of your recovery. When you are at full strength you may resume the regular demands of your daily grind. For most people this is 2 to 4 months after surgery. If you do heavy or physical labor it may be longer.

Once you return to your job, it seems like work will always find you!

65. When can I drive?

It takes a few weeks after surgery before you can drive. Your incision should be well healed and you should recover some of the strength in your operated leg. You should be recovered enough so that a minor impact would not cause damage to your healing wound or new joint.

Most people start driving about 4 weeks after surgery. At first getting in and out of the car may be the hardest thing. It will be difficult to bend your operated hip enough to get through the door. There is more strain on the healing muscles around your hip if you are sitting in a driving position for too long a time. Smaller cars obviously have tighter spaces and pose a greater challenge. On the other hand, the seat in a large SUV may be more comfortable, but getting in may require stepping up on a narrow running board and this may be hard to do.

If your car has an automatic transmission, it will be easier to resume driving if you have had surgery on the left side. This is because you will have normal strength and movement on your right to operate the pedals.

If the right leg has been operated, it will take longer to regain enough strength and control to operate both pedals in the car.

If you drive a manual transmission and have to use a clutch, you will need to have good control of both your right and your left no matter which side has had surgery.

It is important to be cautious. In the first few weeks after surgery, there is a risk of wound disruption or dislocation. Being involved in an accident can cause a major problem even though it is not your fault.

When you resume driving, start slowly. One way to test yourself is to take your car in to an open space when no other cars are around. An example might be the empty parking lot of a shopping center early on a Sunday morning. You will have time to practice and a little more time to react. Practice accelerating and braking until you are sure you have good control. Go for short drives first. You may be uncomfortable sitting in the car with your hip flexed for a long period of time. Try not to get caught in a traffic jam where you are stuck in the car and cannot get out. Wait until your strength increases and your stamina improves.

A temporary handicap parking sticker may be helpful. You can usually obtain one at your local town hall or municipal building. You will need to fill out a form and have it signed by your surgeon.

66. When is it safe to have sex?

The short answer is as soon as everything has healed and you feel comfortable. Usually, this will be 4 to 6 weeks after surgery.

As more people have hip replacement surgery in their thirties, forties, and fifties, this question is asked a lot more often. Of course, there is no right answer.

Once you have had a total hip arthroplasty, it is important not to do anything that would hamper your recovery.

First and foremost, the skin incision and underlying soft tissues around the joint need time to heal. The hip muscles need to regain their strength. Care has to be taken so that the skin incision is not disrupted.

Beyond this, it will take some time for postoperative pain to resolve and time to regain mobility of the joint.

There is still a need to observe dislocation precautions. It takes 3 to 4 months for the lining of the joint, the joint capsule, to heal. Until that time, there is a risk of dislocation. You have to avoid flexing your new hip too much, crossing your legs, twisting movements, and any movement that internally rotates the leg or turns it inward.

Passive positions and positions that avoid pressure on the operated area tend to be more comfortable.

Of course, good communication with your partner is essential. Let your partner know what is comfortable for you and what is not. Everyone heals at a different rate. Some people take longer than others.

Typically, it is about 4 to 6 weeks until you are ready to resume normal relations. If you have any questions, ask your surgeon first! He will be able to tell you when it is safe to resume relations and what precautions should be taken.

67. When can I resume sports? What kind of sports activities are safe?

Many people who have had hip replacement surgery are anxious to resume sports activities. The time to resume sports is when you have fully recovered from surgery.

It is important that you regain the normal tone, strength, and control of the muscles of your lower extremities. This is particularly true of the leg that has just undergone surgery.

While you are having physical therapy for your hip, you should do strengthening exercises for your upper body as well. This will help with your overall return to sports activity.

As your hip gets stronger, advance to distance walking and then swimming. Both of these are safe activities which can improve your overall fitness and increase the strength in your lower extremities. If you are swimming at an indoor pool, you should take extra care not to fall on slippery wet tile surfaces. You should also avoid jumping into the pool or diving in the first few months after surgery. Either of these activities could cause an undue impact on you hip. In some circumstances, they might even cause a dislocation.

In the beginning, try to avoid any activities that would place your hip at risk for injury. When you are fully recovered, you may resume other types of sports activity. Many people who have had hip replacement may safely resume light recreational sports. Examples would be hiking, swimming, jogging, biking, doubles tennis, deep sea diving, and golf. These can maintain your overall level of fitness and enjoyment without putting too much strain on your hip.

Activities with heavy impact, however, will put more pressure on your joint replacement. This might increase long-term wear and lead to eventual loosening or failure of your new hip joint. It is not known how much use or wear and tear will cause long-term failure of an implant. Activities such as high impact aerobics, singles tennis, racquetball, skiing, climbing, surfing, heavy weightlifting, and competitive team sports carry a greater risk.

In particular, sports such as skiing, climbing, or contact sports put you at risk for a fall or a severe twisting injury. This can lead to dislocation of the prosthesis. Dislocation can occur with trauma years after surgery.

While some high level professional athletes such as Bo Jackson of the Chicago White Sox have resumed competitive sports after total hip replacement, they are the exception rather than the rule. Most of these athletes are putting the short-term goals of fame and lucrative professional sports above the long-term future of their hips.

While some high level professional athletes such as Bo Jackson of the Chicago White Sox have resumed competitive sports after total hip replacement, they are the exception rather than the rule.

If you have any questions about what sports are safe after hip surgery, you should ask your doctor. He will tell you what is best and what is safe for your age, activity level, and the condition of your hip. He can also help you if you are working out at a gym and have questions about which exercise machines are safe to use.

After surgery, you want to take care of your new hip and make sure it lasts a long, long time.

Boris K., a patient, says:

I feel like I am a different person—I can take a long walk, I can run, I can jump. I resumed playing tennis, I am taking dance classes now on an advanced level, and nobody notices that I have an artificial hip.

PART NINE

Risks and Complications

How do I know if I have an infection?
How can an infection be diagnosed?

What is a dislocation? What can cause
dislocation?

What other medical complications can happen
from surgery?

More . . .

68. How do I know if I have an infection? How can an infection be diagnosed?

Infection is a known complication of any surgical procedure. Any time you break the skin, such as a scratch, needle puncture, or small cut, there is always a risk of infection. It follows then that a larger surgical wound can also become infected.

The incidence of infection in total joint replacement is just under 1%. The infection can come from local sources, such as the skin and tissues around the wound, or can be blood borne from other sources in the body. If, for example, you have an untreated infection in your urinary tract, it can travel through your blood stream to the prosthetic joint.

A local problem, such as a wound hematoma where fluid sits and becomes infected, can also seed the joint.

Total joint infections can occur in the immediate postoperative period (early) or years down the line (late). Late infections are usually the result of seeding from other parts of the body. A prior infection may also become reactivated. This can occur in individuals who have had previous hip surgery years before their total hip replacement. Even though the old infection seems to be inactive, some bacteria may linger in the bone and cause an infection in a new prosthetic joint. For this reason, it is important to determine if an individual has any history of hip injury or hip surgery that became infected before total hip replacement is considered.

If there is any question, appropriate testing should be done preoperatively to make sure there is no infection.

Some patients, such as those with diabetes mellitus, transplantations, and patients whose immune system is compromised, have a higher risk of infection. There is also a greater risk in patients who have psoriasis and sickle cell disease. Furthermore, the infection rate for joint replacement patients with rheumatoid arthritis is higher than for those with osteoarthritis.

Revision hip procedures have a higher rate of infection than primary hip replacements. There is also a greater risk in cases requiring complex reconstruction and the use of large **allografts**, which are large segments of bone graft taken from freeze-dried cadaver material.

Allograft
Bone that is taken from a cadaver donor and used as a bone graft.

An early postoperative wound infection may first present as swelling, redness or drainage from the wound. The symptoms of a late onset infection might include fever, swelling, and pain either with weight bearing or at rest. There may be redness about the wound, and the wound may begin to open or develop a small sinus. In addition to wound changes, examination will reveal decreased range of motion and pain with movement.

If an infection is suspected, several steps can be taken to make the diagnosis. First, blood studies can be obtained. White blood cells in the body are used to fight infection. An elevated white blood cell count often means that the body has increased the number of white blood cells to fight a new infection. The erythrocyte sedimentation rate (ESR) is a nonspecific test. An elevated ESR, however, is a sign of an active disease process within the body. C-reactive protein is another blood test that when elevated may signal an infection.

X-rays will usually be unremarkable in an early infection. They will show the normal total joint components in place within normal bone. If the infection is chronic, however, bony changes will be seen on x-ray. There may be areas of *lysis* where the bone has been destroyed by infection. The components themselves may change position because they are no longer well seated in bone. A collection of fluid or pus near the bone or the joint may be visible on a CT scan.

If an infection is suspected but there are no changes on plain x-ray, a nuclear study, such as a bone scan or indium scan, may help make the diagnosis. A bone scan will be positive and show any local area of abnormal bone activity within the body. An indium scan is similar to a bone scan but is specific for white blood cell activity and will be positive only if the abnormal activity is due to an infection.

Aspiration is a test that removes fluid from the joint so that it can be tested for bacteria. It is usually done under continuous x-ray or fluoroscopy. A needle is carefully inserted into the joint space, the position of the needle checked on x-ray, then some of the joint fluid is withdrawn through the needle. A specimen is sent to the laboratory so that it can be examined under a microscope and cultured for bacteria. An aspiration can not only tell if an infection is present but can identify the offending organism. This can be helpful in selecting the right antibiotic for treatment.

If pus is obtained on aspiration, it is an obvious sign of infection.

Sometimes, the diagnosis of infection is not clear cut and may be based on a combination of factors. If you have had a hip joint replacement and think that you have developed an infection, contact your doctor immediately. The sooner the diagnosis is made, the sooner treatment may be started. If treatment is started early enough, it may be possible to prevent the infection from becoming more severe and to save the prosthetic joint. If the infection is coming from another part of your body, knowing the source of the infection may help with treatment.

69. How can an infection be treated? How long will I need antibiotics?

All infections require treatment with antibiotics. Most cases also need a surgical procedure.

A superficial infection, that only involves the skin or the layers directly beneath the skin, can sometimes be treated with antibiotics alone. If the infection goes deep in to the joint, then surgery is required to drain the infection and remove the infected tissue.

Antibiotics have to be given intravenously because oral antibiotics are not strong enough and do not provide tissue levels great enough to treat an infected total hip.

If the infection is acute, and is less than 2 weeks old, it can sometimes be treated by a combination of antibiotics and a surgical procedure to wash out or irrigate the wound and remove, or *debride,* any unhealthy tissue. Most total hip infections, however, require more extensive surgery.

The choice of antibiotic depends upon the type of organism that is causing the infection. If surgery is performed, a tissue specimen will be taken and sent to the laboratory for culture. Otherwise, a needle may be inserted in to the hip joint to try to obtain a culture specimen. Bacteria are classified as *gram-positive* or *gram-negative*. The two most common organisms that cause hip infections, *Staph aureus* and *Staph epidermidis*, are both gram-positive. In general gram-positive infections are easier to treat and have a better prognosis than gram-negative infections. Some gram-positive bacteria, such as *methicillin-resistant Staph aureus* (MRSA) and *group D Streptococcus*, are more difficult to treat. Some gram-negative species, such as *enterococcus*, are also difficult.

If you have an infection, your orthopaedic surgeon may ask an infectious disease specialist to assist with your care. He will help your surgeon choose the appropriate antibiotic. At first, treatment is started with a broad spectrum antibiotic, which covers a wide range of organisms. When the culture results have been obtained, an antibiotic that is most effective against the specific organism can be prescribed. This is based on a laboratory test of the organism called *sensitivity*. Some of the most common antibiotics used to treat infections are Ancef, Vancomycin, and Clindamycin.

Intravenous antibiotics need to be given for a period of at least 6 weeks to treat an infected total hip. This is the time required for the antibiotic to reach adequate levels in bone and treat the infection.

In years past, an IV line would have to be replaced every 2 or 3 days. Now a peripherally inserted central catheter (PICC line) can be placed and will last the full 6 weeks. The PICC line is placed as a sterile procedure through a vein in the arm or elbow. It is then passed centrally in to a large vein in the chest called the **superior vena cava**. With proper care, a PICC line can remain in place to give antibiotics for several weeks.

In the past, you had to stay in the hospital while you were having IV antibiotics. Now you can often go home with the line in place and have daily antibiotic injections at an outpatient clinic. The injections can also be given by a visiting nurse who comes to your home. This will allow you to be more functional during your recovery.

Your infectious disease doctor will monitor the doses of antibiotic you are given and check the antibiotic levels in your body. He will make sure you are not having any reaction or side effects to the medication. During treatment, blood tests will be taken to check the white blood cell count, ESR, and C-reactive protein. If these tests become normal again, it is a sign that the infection is improving. Sometimes a repeat needle aspiration may be done and culture specimen obtained. A negative aspiration does not guarantee that the infection is gone, but a positive test means that further treatment is required.

When a hip joint replacement becomes infected, it is important to look for and treat the source of the infection. This may be an infection in another part of the body such as the urinary tract. If the source of the infection is not treated, it can recur in the prosthetic joint.

Infections are harder to treat in patients whose immune system is suppressed, such as transplant patients or patients with HIV.

Most total hip infections will require surgery as part of the treatment. An exception is sometimes made for very elderly or medically debilitated patients in whom the

Superior vena cava

A large vein in the chest which brings blood from the head, neck, arms and chest back to the heart.

infection can be partially treated or suppressed. These patients may live with a chronic infection and need to stay on oral antibiotics for the rest of their lives.

Most healthy patients, however, need surgery in addition to antibiotics as part of their treatment.

70. What kind of surgery is needed to treat an infection?

Almost all total hip infections require surgery. Experience has shown that unless the joint components are removed, the infection cannot be cured. The goal of surgery is to remove all infected tissue and as much of the bacterial contamination as possible. Bacteria are often present at the interface between the components and bone or between cement and bone. Unless the components are removed and the bone cleaned and debrided, the infection will not be cured. Antibiotics do not penetrate well in to these areas and the components themselves can become a focus of the infection.

If there is good fixation, removal of the components may be difficult. If cement is present, it can be hard to separate the cement from bone and remove all of the cement present in the femoral canal or acetabulum. By the same token, if the components have been fixed by bony ingrowth then the metal surfaces have to be carefully separated from the interdigitating bone. This can sometimes result in bone loss as the components are removed.

In the late 1960s and 1970s components were most often left out permanently. It was felt that they could not be reimplanted in the face of infection. Patients were often left with a painful hip and a shortened leg.

With newer antibiotics and better surgical technique, reimplantation is now possible. Most total hip infections are treated with a procedure called **two-stage exchange arthroplasty**.

The components are removed and the joint debrided as the first surgical procedure. Treatment then consists of several weeks of intravenous antibiotics. If blood tests and aspiration are normal and there are no signs of infection, new components may be implanted in the second stage of the procedure. The typical interval between the first and second stage is 6 to 8 weeks.

An antibiotic loaded cement spacer may be placed in the joint between the first and second procedures. The antibiotic, usually Gentamycin, Tobramycin or Vancomycin, will gradually extrude from the cement into the surrounding tissue. The cement spacer can be molded into the shape of a hip joint component. This will prevent contracture of the hip joint while the tissues are healing. It will also permit limited weight bearing. The cement spacer is removed as part of the second stage of the procedure when the new components are implanted.

In some circumstances, a single procedure called **one-stage exchange arthroplasty** can be done. The old components are removed and new components are implanted in a single procedure. Results however are less favorable than with a two-stage procedure.

71. What is DVT? How can it be diagnosed?

DVT means deep vein thrombosis. This occurs when a blood clot forms in one of the deep veins of the calf, thigh, or pelvis.

Two-stage exchange arthroplasty
Treatment for total hip infections where components are removed in a first procedure and new components are reimplanted several weeks later when the infection has cleared.

One-stage exchange arthroplasty
An operation to treat infection where old components are removed and new components are implanted in a single procedure.

DVT is a known complication of hip replacement surgery. The incidence following elective total hip replacement ranges from 3% to 10% even with prophylaxis after surgery.

Some of the risk factors for DVT are:

- Lower extremity fractures
- Elective lower extremity surgery (such as total hip replacement)
- Prolonged bed rest
- Pregnancy
- Birth control pills
- Smoking
- Obesity
- Clotting disorders
- History of DVT or embolic disease
- Malignancy

The greatest risk for DVT is in the first 2 to 10 days after hip surgery. In some cases, it can occur weeks later.

Stasis

When blood sits or pools in a vein and does not flow normally.

The greatest risk for DVT is in the first 2 to 10 days after hip surgery. In some cases, it can occur weeks later.

DVT develops when the circulation or blood flow in one of the deep veins is impaired. The blood becomes stationary and can pool and form clots. Virchow's triad, described in 1856, lists three main factors that cause a clot to form in a vein. These include damage to the vessel wall, blood coagulation, and limited blood flow through the vein or **stasis**. Some surgeons feel that manipulating the leg and retraction of vessels during surgery may be factors that predispose a clot to form.

Phlebitis can be superficial or deep. Clots in superficial veins near the skin are less likely to become large or to migrate. Clots in the larger veins of the calf or thigh are more serious. These clots can break away and travel through the blood stream to cause a clot in the lung or **pulmonary embolus**.

Since hip replacement surgery is associated with a risk of DVT, symptoms or findings that suggest a clot should lead to further investigation. The common symptoms of DVT in the lower leg are pain, swelling, warmth, and tightness or burning.

On physical examination, there is tenderness in a localized area of the calf, swelling, and sometimes warmth or redness. There may be discoloration of the leg or pain with movement of the ankle and knee. A hardness of the vein, or cord, may develop. *Homan's sign*, calf pain when the ankle is flexed with the knee straight, may be present.

The most common test for DVT is an ultrasound or *Doppler* study. This is not painful and does not require x-ray. In a Doppler study an instrument called a *transducer* is placed on the leg and sonic waves are bounced off the deep structures within the leg. These provide images of the vessels and allow the technician to watch the blood flow in the legs. Doppler studies are most effective in the larger veins in the thigh, but can also detect a clot in the calf. A Doppler has the advantage of being risk free. It is not painful and does not require an injection or use of dye.

Venography is done by injecting contrast or dye into the venous system of the leg. It has the disadvantage of requiring radiation exposure and can do damage to the vein itself. Some patients may be allergic to the contrast material. Venography, however, is highly accurate.

Pulmonary embolus
A blood clot in the lung.

165

MRI and MRI venography are evolving techniques that use *gadolinium* instead of iodine contrast. This can be injected through a peripheral vein in the arm and not through the venous system of the leg. It is especially useful for showing clots in the upper thigh or pelvis.

Not all patients with DVT are symptomatic. For this reason, some institutions routinely perform an ultra-sound several days after hip surgery. This can be useful in detecting clots before they become a larger problem.

Most often DVT can be treated and leaves no residual. A small number of patients, however, develop a post-thrombotic syndrome due to permanent damage in the vein. This can lead to chronic pain and swelling in the involved leg.

72. How is a blood clot treated?

Once the diagnosis of DVT is made, treatment needs to be started as soon as possible. The goal of treatment is to prevent the clot in the leg from breaking loose and causing a pulmonary embolus, as well as to ease pain and swelling in the leg. At this point, a specialist in internal medicine or internist usually becomes involved in the treatment.

If DVT occurs in the first few days after surgery, a decision needs to be made as to the level of treatment. This is because aggressive anticoagulation can cause bleeding which leads to a hematoma and wound heal-ing problems. The decision as to treatment is made jointly by the internist and the orthopaedic surgeon.

A small clot in the calf may be treated by observation only or by a combination of observation and no change in the amount of blood thinner. A larger clot in the calf or thigh almost always requires a greater dose of anticoagulation. This usually consists of Heparin given intravenously until the blood thinner reaches an adequate level. Heparin is followed by Warfarin (Coumadin), which is given orally.

Sometimes it is necessary for a patient with DVT to remain at bed rest for several days until he or she is fully anticoagulated. This will help prevent the clot from dislodging and moving to the lung. The surgeon or the internist will decide when it is safe to restart physical therapy.

The duration of treatment following a clot is normally 3 to 6 months. During this time, blood tests will be taken at regular intervals to check the dose of blood thinner. Sometimes the clot will be monitored by follow-up ultrasound studies to make sure that it is resolving.

Patients at very high risk for DVT or who cannot tolerate anticoagulation may be candidates for an inferior vena cava filter. A filter should also be considered in patients who develop a pulmonary embolus despite having been on anticoagulation.

73. What is a pulmonary embolus?

A pulmonary embolus is a blood clot that goes to the lungs. In hip surgery, it is the result of clots forming in the deep veins of the legs and moving into the venous system of the body. It is not clear what causes the clots to break loose. When they do, they travel upward in the body through a large vein called the *inferior vena cava*. They pass through the right side of the heart into the *pulmonary artery*. They are then pumped through the pulmonary artery or into its branches and reach the lungs.

When a clot reaches a part of the lung, it causes a pulmonary embolus. This means that the blood supply to that part of the lung is blocked and cannot transport oxygen.

When a clot reaches a part of the lung, it causes a pulmonary embolus. This means that the blood supply to that part of the lung is blocked and cannot transport oxygen. After a pulmonary embolus, you have less oxygen in your body.

A pulmonary embolus can be either a single clot or multiple emboli. If a large portion of a lung is affected, the consequences can be severe. It can lead to lack of oxygen in your body and damage to your circulatory system and other organs. It can sometimes be fatal.

Most times, a pulmonary embolus occurs as an acute event in the first 3 weeks after surgery. The main symptom is sudden acute chest pain. There can be rapid breathing and shortness of breath. There can also be heart palpitations. Shortness of breath may be accompanied by coughing and sometimes *hemoptysis,* or coughing up blood. There will be an increase in heart rate or pulse and the skin may become pale.

A small device attached to your finger, a *pulse oximeter,* will show a decreased amount of oxygen in your bloodstream.

In a few cases, a pulmonary embolus can present as a silent event. Patients may have little more than a fever, dizziness, and a sense of not feeling well. When this happens, a high index of suspicion is needed to make the diagnosis.

The test used to make the diagnosis of pulmonary embolus is a *spiral CT scan.* This is a special type of CT scan where the scanner rotates around your body to create special three-dimensional images. It is highly accurate in diagnosing a blood clot in your lungs.

The treatment of a pulmonary embolus is similar to the treatment for a blood clot in the legs. Rapid anti-coagulation is started with intravenous heparin. This is switched to Coumadin by mouth once an adequate level of anticoagulation has been reached. Coumadin is continued for several months. Patients are also given oxygen and other forms of pulmonary support.

If a patient is at high risk for further emboli, a filter or umbrella can be placed in the inferior vena cava.

Physical therapy can be resumed when a patient is medically stable and adequate levels of anticoagulation have been reached.

Pulmonary embolism is one of the reasons for giving blood thinners after hip surgery. Most often it is a treatable event that delays recovery for only a short period of time. In rare cases the consequences can be serious and this is one of the main complications of hip replacement surgery.

74. What is a dislocation? What can cause dislocation?

Dislocation of a hip replacement occurs when the ball of the hip comes out of the socket.

For a total hip, this means that the prosthetic femoral head comes out of the prosthetic acetabulum. For a bipolar replacement, it means that the prosthetic bipolar head comes out of the normal hip joint socket.

Dislocation is a known complication of total hip arthroplasty. The overall incidence has been quoted as anywhere from 0.3% to 10% depending upon the study.

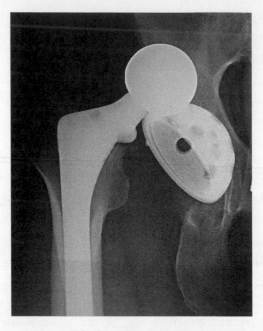

Figure 29 X-ray of a total hip dislocation. The ball has come out of the socket.

Some reviews have shown that women are more likely to dislocate than men in the postoperative period. Other research has suggested that older people dislocate more than younger people.

Beyond this, there is some evidence that total hip replacements done as treatment for an acute fracture are at greater risk for dislocation than replacements done for arthritis.

When total hip replacement is performed, incisions are made in the soft tissues that hold the natural hip in place in the socket. Some of the muscles and ligaments around the joint are divided. The thick lining of the joint, the *hip joint capsule* is also divided and retracted. As a result, there is less soft tissue after surgery to protect the hip from coming out of the socket.

The diameters of the new femoral head and socket are different than the normal hip. A normal femoral head is typically 43 mm or greater. The femoral heads used in total hip replacements have a diameter of 22–36 mm. The smaller size makes it much easier for the prosthetic femoral head to come out of the socket.

Accordingly, you should take precautions against dislocation after a total hip replacement until the ligaments and capsule around the joint have had a chance to heal.

Most dislocations occur within the first 3 or 4 months after surgery, but dislocation can occur at any time, even years down the line. If the soft tissues which hold the hip in place are badly damaged, the dislocations may recur and cause a chronic instability of the hip.

There are many reasons for dislocation. It is felt, however, that most dislocations are multifactorial or due to several causes at once.

Some patient groups are known to be at higher risk for dislocation. For example, patients who have neuromuscular disease, such as parkinsonism or muscular dystrophy, may have some loss of voluntary muscle control and thus may not be able to prevent the hip from coming out of the socket. Similarly, patients who have cognitive problems, senility, or dementia will be unable to follow the normal precautions and prevent dislocation. Alcoholism is associated with a high dislocation rate.

An unexpected fall or injury can also cause the hip to come out of the socket.

Sometimes the cause of dislocation can be attributed to soft tissue problems. If there is not enough soft tissue tension in the system, the muscles may be loose and allow the joint to come out of place. Modular components which increase the soft tissue tension, but not the length of the prosthesis, can sometimes prevent this problem.

The position of the components may also play a role. If the acetabular component is tilted too far in one direction, the femoral head may be uncovered when a patient is in a walking or sitting position. This can lead to dislocation.

In other situations, the components themselves are the issue. Some components, such as "skirted" femoral heads or acetabular liners with elevated rims, can cause impingement and actually help to push the hip out of the socket.

Overall, it is felt that hip replacements with larger femoral heads may be more stable and less likely to dislocate.

Dislocation can be related to long-term wear of the components. If the polyethylene liner of the socket has worn thin, the femoral head may be more likely to slip out. If there has been subsidence of the femoral component, there may be less soft tissue tension and a tendency for the hip to dislocate.

Most often, the dislocation is the result of a combination of factors. Dislocations in the first few months after surgery have a better prognosis and are less likely to develop chronic instability than those which occur later on. It is therefore important to observe dislocation precautions in the immediate postoperative period. Your orthopaedic surgeon along with the team of nurses and physical therapists at the hospital will give you a list of dos and don'ts to help protect your hip from dislocating. It is important to take the proper precautions in the first 3 to 4 months after surgery.

If dislocation does occur, a **reduction** procedure will be needed to put the hip back in place.

Reduction

A procedure to put a dislocated hip back in place either by manipulation or open surgery.

75. If I have a dislocation will I need to have more surgery?

Most dislocations occur as an acute sudden event and are immediately obvious. Typically, a dislocation will result from an abnormal twist and fall.

The hip and leg become acutely painful. Often the leg will appear to be shortened and rotated. If a dislocation occurs, you will have difficulty moving your hip and your leg. You will be unable to stand or bear weight.

For this reason, most dislocations are put back into place a short time after they occur.

If you think you have injured or dislocated your hip, you should remain in place and seek immediate help. You should contact your surgeon and go to the hospital emergency room.

At the hospital, you will be examined either by an emergency room physician or by your own orthopaedic surgeon. Since dislocations are very painful, most are put back in place within a few hours after they occur.

A procedure to put a dislocated hip back into place is called a *reduction*. A closed reduction means that the hip is put back into place by manipulation without having to reopen the incision.

Most dislocations can be reduced closed. Frequently, the procedure can be done in an emergency room setting with either intravenous sedation or with light general anesthesia.

In some circumstances, more anesthesia and complete muscle relaxation are required. When this happens, the procedure is done under general anesthesia in an operating room. Sometimes the surgeon may use a special type of x-ray called *fluoroscopy* to help with the procedure. Fluoroscopy involves a continuous x-ray that allows the surgeon to monitor the position of the femoral head as he attempts to put it back in the socket.

When the hip joint is reduced, there will be a sudden palpable *clunk* which is evident to all in the operating room. The surgeon will then obtain an x-ray to confirm that the hip is reduced. He will place the hip through a range of motion to check and make sure that the hip is stable. Most closed reductions are done by flexing the hip and gently rotating it back into position.

If the hip cannot be reduced by closed manipulation an *open reduction* will be required. An open reduction is a procedure where a surgical incision is made (most often through the previous surgical scar) and the hip joint is exposed. The dislocated head and the socket are identified. Any soft tissue, such as muscle or capsule that is blocking the reduction is removed. The hip joint is then put directly back into place by the surgeon. After the joint has been reduced, the surgeon will place the hip through a careful range of motion. He will want to evaluate the stability of the joint in every position.

If he feels that the joint is unstable and likely to dislocate again, he may want to change or remove some of the components. If the joint feels loose, he may choose to put a longer head on the femur and thereby increase the length. This will create greater tension in the muscles and make it harder for the hip to come out of place. He may choose to substitute a new polyethylene liner for the socket that has an elevated wall or rim which acts as a barrier to dislocation. If he feels that the angle of the socket or sometimes the femur needs to be changed, he may remove the entire component and place a new one at a different angle. It is not uncommon for a surgeon to change the angle or anteversion of the prosthetic socket.

Since many total hip components are modular, part of the component may be removed without having to disturb the component's fixation to bone. This is true of the femoral head and neck and the polyethylene lining of the socket.

In more difficult cases, the surgeon may chose to tighten some of the muscles around the hip by doing a procedure called **trochanteric osteotomy**. In this procedure, the abductor muscles which insert on the greater trochanter of the hip are advanced further down the femur and thus tightened. Greater muscle tension will help to keep the hip joint in place.

In some cases, a partial or bipolar replacement will be more stable than a total hip. The prosthetic socket is then removed and a larger or bipolar head is attached to the femur.

In extreme cases, a *constrained* acetabular component is used to hold the femoral head in place. A constrained component has a special ring on the outside which locks in the femoral head. This type of component, however,

Trochanteric osteotomy

A technique where the greater trochanter is detached from the femur and re-attached lower down to tighten muscles and create greater stability.

175

limits range of motion and is not suitable for young, active, or high-demand patients. Constrained cups have a high failure rate and are used for salvage cases.

After closed reduction, most patients are treated by observation and care to avoid positions that cause dislocation. Sometimes the surgeon may recommend an abduction pillow for sleeping or may prescribe limited or protected weight bearing while the hip is healing.

Many surgeons order a special dislocation brace that patients wear for 3 to 6 months following reduction. This type of brace limits flexion and abduction and protects the hip from those positions that would tend to cause dislocation.

While open surgery is not common for dislocations, it is sometimes necessary particularly in those patients who experience multiple dislocation episodes.

76. What is leg length inequality? How does it happen?

Leg length inequality
When one leg is longer or shorter than the other.

Leg length inequality means one leg is longer or shorter than the other. Very often your legs are not equal before surgery and it is hard to make them equal afterward. Many factors come into play besides the actual length or height of your femur.

You should tell your surgeon if one of your legs feels shorter than the other.

Preoperative evaluation is very important. You should tell your surgeon if one of your legs feels shorter than the other. Usually, this is the side with your bad hip. Your leg may feel shorter because the joint space has decreased and your femoral head has flattened and lost height. You may have also developed a flexion contracture which makes it impossible to fully straighten your leg. This too can make your leg feel shorter.

For exam
side o
is

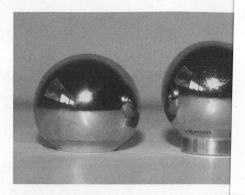

**Figure 30   Different neck lengths allow the su
joint more stable.**

Your surgeon will measure your leg lengths when he does
his physical examination. It is important to tell him,
however, if your legs feel short or long even if his measurements seem different than what you feel. He will take
this into account when he is doing your surgery.

Your orthopaedic surgeon will measure both *true leg
length* and *apparent leg length*. The true leg length is
the measurement of your leg without regard to your
spine or pelvis. It is measured from a fixed point on
your pelvis called the *anterior superior iliac spine* to the
inner bone of your ankle called the *medial malleolus*.
Thus true lengths are measured from separate points
on each leg.

Apparent leg length is measured from your *umbilicus*
(belly button) to the medial malleolus on each side. It
is measured from the same upper point on your body to
each leg. If your pelvis is not level, then the apparent
leg length will be greater on one side than the other
even though true leg lengths may be equal. This is
important to know because your leg lengths may feel
different when you are standing or walking, even
though the absolute measurement of your legs is equal.

ple, if you have a curvature of your spine, one your pelvis may be higher than the other. This called *pelvic obliquity*. Your leg may feel shorter because one side of your pelvis is higher. There may also be *pelvic tilt* or rotation that can affect the apparent length of your legs.

One way to evaluate this is to do a standing block test. In this test your surgeon will place blocks of different heights under your shorter leg until your pelvis is level.

Overcorrecting an apparent but not a true inequality can lead to back pain and make you feel uncomfortable.

Measurements are not always exact. In obese patients the measurement points can be hard to locate. Sometimes, special x-rays to measure the leg lengths can be helpful.

Your surgeon will take any leg length differences into account when he plans your surgery. He may place a template of different size and length hip components over your x-ray to see which fits best and which provides any needed correction.

It is not always possible at surgery to make leg lengths perfectly equal. Lengths may be hard to judge on the operating table.

Several methods are available in the operating room, but they are not always exact. The surgeon may take measurements from one point to another, both before and after placement of the components. This will determine if there is any difference. He may also do a side to side comparison of the operative to the nonoperative leg. Sometimes, he may take an x-ray.

None of these measurements however are precise.

On the operating table, the surgeon can affect lengths by placing the femoral stem higher or lower. He can also adjust lengths by placing a longer or shorter head-neck component on top of the femoral stem. This gives the surgeon some flexibility in making adjustments or corrections.

In some cases, it may be necessary to lengthen the operative leg in order to make the hip stable. Increasing the height or length a small amount will lengthen the soft tissues around the joint. This will make it harder for the femoral head to come out of place.

Most patients will tolerate a small amount of shortening or lengthening and never even notice the difference. Your body can adjust to small differences without difficulty. It may, however, take 3 to 6 months for your body to fully accommodate. This means that for a time after surgery your leg lengths may feel different even though a good correction has been made.

If both of your hips are bad, then your operated hip will feel longer after surgery. The difference will be corrected when your other hip is replaced.

If your legs feel unequal after surgery, a shoe lift may help. Typically the operative side is longer and you will need to wear the lift on the opposite shoe. This will make you feel more comfortable and make it easier to walk. The size of the lift should be determined by trial and error. You should wear whatever makes you feel best. There is no right or wrong size, only individual comfort.

Too much lengthening can cause problems on the operative site. It can cause back pain or sciatic symptoms, such as pain, numbness, or even weakness of the muscles of the lower leg. Talk to your orthopaedic surgeon if you have any of these symptoms.

77. What is heterotopic ossification?

Heterotopic ossification, or **ectopic bone** as it is sometimes known, is abnormal bone that forms in the soft tissues around bone or near a joint.

Heterotopic ossification

Abnormal bone that forms in the soft tissues around a bone or near a joint.

Bone formation in the soft tissues is a known complication of hip replacement surgery or any surgery around the hip. It is not known what causes the bone to form or why it happens after joint replacement.

Heterotopic ossification (H.O.) can occur after joint replacement, after fracture repair, or sometimes after fractures that are treated nonoperatively. It forms around larger joints, such as the hip, knee, shoulder, or elbow. It is known to occur after neurologic events, such as stroke or spinal cord injury, and is sometimes seen in head injury patients who have orthopaedic injuries as well. Beyond this, H.O. can develop in patients who have had severe burns.

The exact cause of H.O. is not clear. It may represent the body's attempt to repair damage after an injury. If the soft tissues around the bone or joint are injured, the body may recognize the injury as a fracture and respond by forming new bone. This may be true if damage occurs to structures close to bone, such as the lining of the bone, the **periosteum**, or to the joint capsule. Injury to these structures may generate an innate healing response and cause bone to form.

Periosteum

The outer lining tissue on the surface of bone.

Basic precursor cells or *mesenchymal* cells may be released or may become active in the tissues. These cells may then

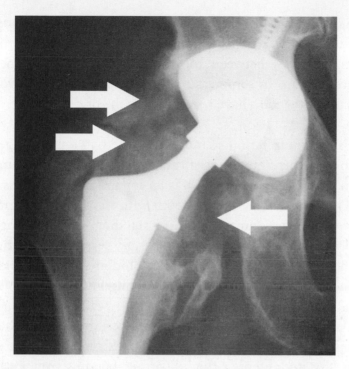

Figure 31 X-ray of a total hip that has developed heterotopic ossification after surgery. A large amount of cloudy white bone (arrows) is bridging the space between the femur and the acetabulum.

give rise to *osteoblasts* which can form bone cells or *osteocytes*. This may be very similar to the type of physiologic reaction that occurs after a fracture.

After hip replacement surgery, the extra or ectopic bone forms in the abductor muscles.

Only a small percentage of patients with H.O. are symptomatic. Most often H.O. is noted in the soft tissues on routine follow-up x-rays after hip replacement. The amount of bone formation is small and usually does not interfere with function. It is an incidental x-ray finding only.

181

Some patients with H.O. do have symptoms. These are patients with advanced disease where dense bone is seen in the space between the top of the femur and the acetabulum. In some cases, it may appear as if the two sides of the joint have been fused by the bridging bone.

Pain and limitation of motion are the two main symptoms of heterotopic ossification. At first there is pain in the joint because H.O. is an inflammatory process. The pain may be present both with movement and at rest. It may occur with sitting, standing, or even lying down. Inflammatory symptoms are best treated with modified activity and NSAIDs. Indomethacin is the most widely used NSAID for treating H.O.

As the process continues, stiffness or limitation of the involved joint develops. In the hip, this may cause difficulty straightening the leg, sitting, bending over, getting up from a chair, or getting in and out of a car. Stiffness in the hip may place additional stress on nearby joints, such as the spine and knee. It may result in lower back pain because movement in the spine has to compensate for the hip.

The process begins and patients are symptomatic well before changes are seen on x-ray. This is because bone cannot be seen on x-ray until it starts to calcify. By then the process has already started and cannot be reversed.

Patients at risk for H.O. following elective hip replacement are those who have had a proliferative type of osteoarthritis with extra bone formation in and around the joint. This is more common in men than women. Patients who developed H.O. after previous trauma to the hip are also at risk when they undergo elective hip replacement. Other risk groups include those who have hypertrophic bone forming conditions, such as Paget's disease or ankylosing spondylitis.

Heterotopic ossification cannot always be prevented, but prophylaxis is indicated after hip surgery for patients who are at high risk.

These patients are often given a single dose of external radiation to the area around the hip. This may be combined with an oral NSAID like indomethacin. The NSAID may be given for a period of up to 6 weeks. Since the bone forming reaction occurs right after surgery, prophylaxis is given within the first 5 days after the procedure.

Surgery to remove the extra bone is rarely necessary. H.O. may be painful for up to 12 months after the hip replacement procedure due to inflammation. Surgery is not done until 12 to 24 months afterward, when new bone formation has stopped. At this point, a bone scan will show no bone forming activity in the region of the hip. A blood test called *alkaline phosphatase* can also be used to measure bone activity.

Surgery is done when a patient cannot tolerate the loss of motion, when loss of motion interferes with daily activity, or when secondary pain develops in areas such as the lumbar spine. In this setting, surgery may be done to remove the ectopic bone.

The surgical procedure involves isolating the bone and dissecting it away from the adjacent muscle and soft tissues. Sometimes the extra bone heals directly to the femur or acetabulum and needs to be separated. The point where normal bone ends and heterotopic bone begins may be hard to identify.

This procedure may have a higher blood loss and a higher incidence of nerve and vascular complications than routine hip surgery. The deep soft tissue structures of the hip are bound up in bone and hard to identify. After surgery there may be a short-term weakness of the muscles around the hip.

After removal of heterotopic bone, motion in the hip joint may improve but may not return to normal. For this reason, surgery is only done for those people who have a severe limitation of function.

78. Can fractures occur during surgery? How can they be treated?

Fractures during surgery are an unusual but treatable complication. The overall incidence of intraoperative fractures is less than 1%.

Fractures are often the result of reaming or press fitting components into soft or osteoporotic bone. Even though care is taken, the bone can crack as the components are impacted. Fractures may also occur through abnormal or pathologic bone, such as in tumor or Paget's disease.

Most intraoperative fractures are benign and are noted only on postoperative x-rays. They appear as a single nondisplaced fracture line near one of the components. These fractures require no treatment except protected weight bearing for a few weeks until healing occurs. Other times, weight bearing may be permitted, and the normal postoperative regimen does not need to be changed at all.

More serious intraoperative fractures can be treated during surgery by using different components or additional fixation.

If the fracture is in the femur, a longer femoral stem might be used to bypass the fracture. Circular cables may be placed around the bone to hold it together. If the fracture occurs in the region of the greater trochanter, a special trochanteric plate and cables can be used to bring the trochanter back to its normal position. A bone graft can sometimes be added to stimulate healing.

On the acetabular side, fractures are treated with a combination of cement, bone graft, or a larger acetabular component that will fix to the edges of the socket.

Most fractures, if recognized and treated during surgery, do not affect the ultimate outcome of the procedure.

In a resurfacing procedure, fractures of the femoral neck may occur in the first few months after surgery. This is because the femoral neck is affected by the reaming of the femoral head needed to fit the femoral component. Fractures after resurfacing are treated by conversion to a conventional total hip arthroplasty.

Fractures around the components can also happen years after surgery. These are called **periprosthetic fractures**. They are usually the result of trauma, such as a fall. Periprosthetic fractures require surgery to stabilize the fracture and sometimes revision of the total hip components.

Periprosthetic fracture

A fracture which occurs around or near a prosthetic component.

79. Can there be injuries to nerves and vessels around the hip?

Problems with nerves and vessels are more likely to happen in difficult revision cases than in first time primary hip replacements.

Most nerve problems after hip surgery are due to pressure or traction. During surgery, instruments called *retractors* are placed in the wound to help the surgeon see the main operating field. They keep the overlying tissue layers away from the hip joint. If a retractor is placed near a nerve for too long, the nerve may be stretched or irritated. Loss of sensation or movement in the area supplied by the nerve can result.

The two main nerves near the hip joint during a total hip replacement are the *femoral nerve* and the *sciatic nerve*. The femoral nerve is in the front of the thigh, the sciatic nerve in the back. Sciatic nerve problems are more common than femoral. The sciatic nerve divides into two branches, the *tibial* and *peroneal*, and it is the peroneal branch that is most often affected.

Nerve injuries present as pain or numbness, but there can be loss of movement. If the peroneal nerve is injured, weakness of the muscles that raise or *dorsiflex* the ankle and toes can cause a foot drop. Femoral nerve problems affect the front of the thigh and the muscles that straighten the knee.

Nerve injuries happen more often in cases where there is unusual anatomy, such as DDH or when the leg is lengthened. In revision cases, the nerves may be encased in scar and hard to identify.

Most, but not all, nerve problems will improve with time and observation. Some regain only partial function or no function at all. Surgery is needed only if there is a direct injury to the nerve or there is a fluid collection causing pressure around the nerve.

Fortunately, there are hardly ever any injuries to the arteries and veins around the hip during hip replacement surgery. If they do happen it may be necessary for your orthopaedic surgeon to consult a vascular surgeon.

80. What other medical complications can happen from surgery?

In addition to blood clots and pulmonary embolism, there are other medical complications that can happen from hip replacement surgery. Most medical complications are minor. They result in little or no increase to your hospital stay and have no effect on the overall time of your recovery. Most are easily treated and resolve quickly.

Fever is common after hip replacement surgery. It is usually the body's reaction to the trauma of the procedure or to bleeding within the tissues. Most orthopaedic surgeons consider a temperature below 100° to be normal during the postoperative period. A postoperative fever will resolve in 2 or 3 days. If the temperature persists above 101°, it may be a sign of an infection in another part of the body such as the lungs or urinary tract. A fever can also be a sign of a drug reaction.

Like fever, anemia is common after surgery. This is due to the blood loss incurred during the surgical procedure. Anemia can sometimes cause low blood pressure, or *hypotension*. It is easily treated by giving a blood transfusion, sometimes with the patient's own autologous blood.

Allergies to medications can present as a rash or itching over the body. An allergic reaction can be treated by stopping the medication and giving a drug like *Benadryl* that will relieve the allergic symptoms. In addition to allergies, medications can have side effects.

For pain medications, these might include nausea and constipation.

Since pain medications affect the nervous system, they can sometimes slow down the muscles that control the urinary tract or intestines. In the urinary tract, you can go into retention; you are unable to void. This is treated by placement of a tube or catheter. The catheter is normally removed after 2 or 3 days.

In the intestines, relaxation of the muscles can lead to *paralytic ileus*. This means your intestines stop working for a short period of time and your abdomen becomes bloated or distended. Like urinary retention, it usually resolves spontaneously after 2 or 3 days.

As with any other major surgical procedure, more serious medical complications can develop after hip replacement. The stress of surgery can affect all the major systems of your body. Serious medical complications include heart failure or arrhythmia, stroke, kidney failure, and pneumonia. Fortunately, most of these events are rare. If they do occur, they will require more extensive treatment and consultation with the appropriate medical specialist.

PART TEN

Revisions and Fractures

When is revision surgery necessary?

How do I know if my hip has loosened?

Are there greater risks from revision surgery?

More . . .

81. When is revision surgery necessary?

While most arthroplasties will last for many years, some will require a **revision** procedure during the patient's lifetime. A revision is a procedure that is done to replace one or more parts of the original total hip arthroplasty.

Revision

A second surgical procedure that is done to replace one or more parts of the original hip replacement.

Years ago, total hip arthroplasties were mostly done in elderly patients. Now, more and more primary total hip replacements are being done in younger patients. Many patients have total hip arthroplasty in their forties or even their thirties! This means that the hip arthroplasty will have to last for a long time in the life of the patient. Since these patients are younger, they are more active and they place higher demand on their hip replacements. The hip arthroplasty will undergo more wear for an extended period of time. For this reason, revision total hip surgery is becoming more common.

There are several reasons why revision surgery may be required:

1. When components loosen

   Components are held in place in bone either by cement or by bony ingrowth. If the bond between the component and the bone changes, the component can loosen. Osteolysis can cause thinning of the bone and the layer of cement or the cement mantle becomes loose. The cement itself may even fracture.

2. When components fail or break

   The earliest designs of femoral stems were subject to fatigue failure and sometimes even to fracture. Fortunately, with newer designs, component fracture is rarely seen.

Polyethylene wear, or wear of the lining inside the socket, is another cause of failure. When this happens, the metal ball of the femoral component may no longer be contained, and the hip may become unstable. In a few cases, fracture of a ceramic femoral head can also occur. This happens because the material is very hard and brittle. When a component breaks or fails, revision is always necessary.

3. When an event occurs that disturbs the fixation to bone

A fracture around the components (periprosthetic fracture) usually requires a revision procedure because the fracture disrupts the fixation of the component to the bone. Most often this occurs around the stem of the femoral component, but it can happen in other areas. Sometimes the joint replacement will have to be revised in order to provide stable fixation of the fracture.

Infection is another event that can create a need for revision. When an infection occurs in a prosthetic joint, some of the bone tissue that holds the components in place may be destroyed. The components may become loose and have to be replaced.

In other situations, one or more of the prosthetic components may settle into the bone. On the acetabular side, the cup may gradually settle deeper into the pelvis and cause a protrusio. On the femoral side, the stem component may settle into the femoral canal. This is called *subsidence*.

4. When the hip is unstable

If the hip has dislocated several times, the hip is said to be unstable and revision is necessary. Revision surgery for dislocation aims to correct the cause of the instability. This may mean revision of one or both sides of the arthroplasty. The angle of a component may need to be changed to make the joint more stable. Another option might be to increase the neck length of the femoral component to add more muscle tension and stability to the system.

Recent data shows that instability is the most common diagnosis for patients undergoing revision surgery followed by mechanical loosening.

82. How do I know if my hip has loosened?

Loosening means that one or both of the hip implants is no longer securely fixed to bone.

The diagnosis of loosening is based on symptoms, physical examination, and radiologic studies such as x-ray, arthrogram, or bone scan.

Many patients will have x-ray findings that suggest loosening several years after surgery. These can take the form of **lucent lines** that surround either the component or the cement mantle. Often lucent lines are just x-ray findings, and patients will have no symptoms.

Lucent lines

Thin, clear lines seen on x-ray between a component and bone or between cement and bone that may indicate component loosening.

Pain is the most common symptom of loosening. The onset may be either sudden or gradual, and pain may begin after a fall or an event that triggers the loosening. Patients may have pain both with activity or just sitting. Sometimes the pain is tolerable, but other times patients cannot bear weight. A patient who is able to walk may require a cane or crutches for support. Other symptoms of loosening may be more mechanical, such as clicking or a sense that a component is moving. If the hip is unstable, patients may feel that the joint is coming out of place, particularly when they are sitting or flexing the hip.

Physical examination may show some tenderness about the hip, but the most common finding is groin and thigh pain with movement. As the surgeon flexes and rotates the hip, the hip becomes painful and reproduces the symptoms. The leg may appear shorter than it has been and it may be turned inward or outward. A rotational deformity occurs because the stem of the component has rotated within the shaft of the femur. If the hip is unstable, a mechanical clicking or clunking may be noted with certain movements.

If loosening is suspected, further studies may need to be done.

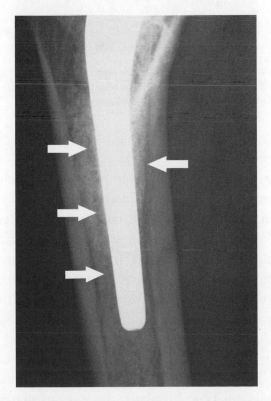

Figure 32   A femoral stem in normal position in a femoral canal. A normal cement pattern (arrows) is seen between the stem and bone.

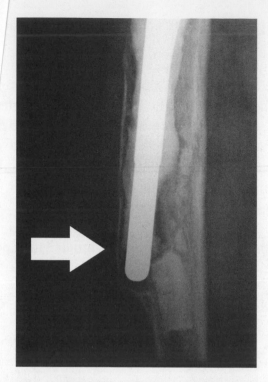

Figure 33 **A loosened femoral stem. The femur has broken away from the cement and the tip is pushing against the edge of the bone (arrow). The outer surface of the bone, the cortex, has become very thin.**

The diagnosis of loosening can most often be made on plain x-ray. Thin clear *lucent lines* may be present between the component and bone or between the cement and bone. When these occur, it is often a sign that the component is separating from the bone. Osteolysis, thinning of the bone, may result in areas next to the prosthesis. An x-ray will show a clear space within the substance of the bone.

Shifting of the components can also be a sign of loosening. The acetabular component may rotate and change its position. Similarly, the stem can change its angle in the shaft or can settle and subside.

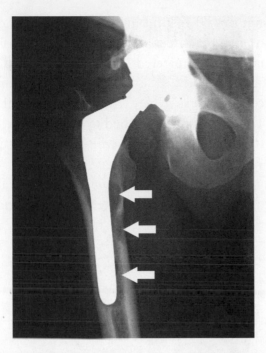

Figure 34   Loosening due to thinning of the bone or osteolysis (arrows).

When the polyethylene liner of the acetabulum is worn or loose the ball of the femur will no longer appear centered in the acetabular component.

If there is any question, an arthrogram can be done. An arthrogram is done by a radiologist. Dye is injected into the joint that can be seen on an x-ray. If the dye fills the space between the component and bone, it is one sign that there is loosening of the component. An arthrogram can also be used to obtain a specimen of joint fluid to see if there is an infection. The fluid can be removed from the joint and sent to the laboratory. There it is both examined under a microscope and cultured for bacteria. A positive culture means that further evaluation and treatment are necessary for infection. A surgical procedure to clean out the infection and sometimes remove the components may be required.

A *bone scan* can be helpful in making the diagnosis of either loosening or infection. In a bone scan, radiosensitive material is injected intravenously and goes throughout the body. It is rapidly cleared from the body except in areas where there is abnormal bony activity. The material is absorbed by osteoblasts, which are cells that make bone, and will show on a scan. If there is new bone activity, it may be a sign of either loosening or infection. An *Indium scan* is like a bone scan but is more specific for white blood cells and thus for infection.

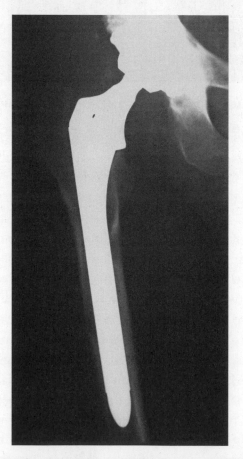

Figure 35   Revision of previous case with longer stem prosthesis extending below the defects in the bone.

All of these studies are helpful in diagnosing the factors that may require revision surgery for loosening or infection.

83. Is a revision procedure more difficult than a regular total hip? Does it take longer?

Most revision surgeries are more difficult than the first time or primary total hip arthroplasty.

After a surgical procedure has been performed, scar tissue forms within the body. The scar tissue is thicker and harder than normal muscle or capsular tissue. When scar tissue forms, the normal anatomic planes between the various structures are obscured. It is therefore more difficult to identify the important anatomy and the surgical exposure is harder. Care has to be taken because structures such as the sciatic nerve may be encased in scar and not easily identified. Beyond this, the presence of scar tissue can make exposure of the components difficult.

More tissue has to be divided or released in a revision procedure to allow for exposure and dislocation of the hip joint. This needs to be done so that the components can be well visualized and removed or revised as necessary.

In a simple revision procedure, only one component may need to be changed. Since some of the components are modular, the revision procedure may take the form of a simple exchange of one polyethylene liner for another. It may also be a simple exchange of one femoral head for another with a longer neck. Sometimes either the entire acetabular component—polyethylene liner and metal backing—or the entire femoral component—stem and modular head—may need to be removed.

In more complex revision cases, both femoral and acetabular components are removed and larger revision components are inserted.

In some cases, a porous backed component that has been fixed by bony ingrowth may need to be separated from bone. Other times, cement may need to be separated from bone and removed from the medullary canal of the femur. This can be a long and tedious process. The cement needs to be carefully separated while doing as little damage as possible to the remaining healthy bone.

Revision procedures require special tools to accomplish these tasks. Long handled chisels and osteotomes are needed to reach deep into the femoral canal. High speed cement drills are also used within the canal to separate cement from bone. Ultrasound is another effective tool for cement removal. The ultrasonic waves break down the cement and help preserve the bone.

On the acetabular side, special rounded chisels that match the diameter of the acetabulum can be used to separate the spherical surface of the component from the underlying bone. This is done in such a way so as to minimize the amount of bone that is removed with a component.

Revision surgery requires special techniques which are most often not necessary in primary total hip replacement. Removal of cement often poses the greatest difficulty. The cement forms a long tube within the medullary canal of the bone. At revision surgery, the

Revision surgery requires special techniques which are most often not necessary in primary total hip replacement.

stem of the femoral component is loose or can be easily tapped out. The long column of cement, however, is embedded, and the portions that are not loose are well fixed to bone. If the cement column is very long, wider exposure may be necessary. In some cases, the cement may extend 5 or 6 inches from the joint into the medullary canal. It often cannot be reached from above. A section of bone must be removed from the femur to expose the cement that is more distal.

In another technique, a longer cut in the bone called an **extended trochanteric osteotomy** exposes the whole tube of cement. This involves cutting a long section of the femur for several inches to provide greater exposure. When this is done, the osteotomy has to be repaired. Special cables or a metal plate and cables are placed around the bone to bring the bone back together over the new femoral component. A bone graft, in the form of a strut, may be used to support the repair or to reinforce thin bone. Sometimes, smaller chips or fragments of bone are compressed in the medullary canal by a technique called **impaction grafting**. In this technique, a layer of bone is placed within the canal to reinforce the bone that is already present.

Similarly, a bone graft may be used in the acetabulum to fill any bony defect.

All of these techniques may be used individually or combined, depending on the nature of the case. Plain x-rays or fluoroscopy are sometimes used to monitor the position of the instruments as the cement is removed.

Removal of cement and well-fixed components during a revision procedure must be done carefully. Otherwise, there is a risk of fracture of the femur or the acetabulum.

Extended trochanteric osteotomy

A technique used in revision surgery where a cut is made in the greater trochanter and femoral shaft to expose the inside of the femoral canal.

Impaction grafting

A procedure where bone chips are packed inside the femoral canal to provide reinforcement for the bone before the prosthesis is inserted.

Since the anatomy is more complex, reconstruction of the bone and trial fitting of the components may take longer than normal. Time may also be spent placing bone grafts and repairing the osteotomy. Beyond this, a revision procedure will require a longer surgical incision and this will take longer to close. Overall, the time required for revision procedure is usually longer than normal.

84. Are special components required for a revision procedure?

When revision procedures involve loss of bone, specialized components are necessary to fill the defects and add additional structure and stability. Most revision components are readily available as off-the-shelf items. Other times, custom components must be ordered and manufactured to fit the particular anatomic defect or situation.

Calcar replacement

A special larger body prosthesis that is used to fill the space on the femoral neck if the calcar is worn down or missing.

On the femoral side, the inside of the femoral neck, the calcar, is frequently worn down or missing. For this reason, it is sometimes necessary to use a **calcar replacement** to fill the space on the femoral neck. Usually, the stem length on a revision femoral component is longer than that used on a primary arthroplasty. This allows more fixation in the lower or distal part of the femur.

Some components add an additional degree of modularity. There are separate components for the stem, the body, and the neck. These allow the revision femoral component to match the size in each part of the femur. In addition, the rotation, or *version*, of the neck may be adjusted to provide greater stability. Frequently revision femoral components will have greater neck lengths to make up for the lost bone.

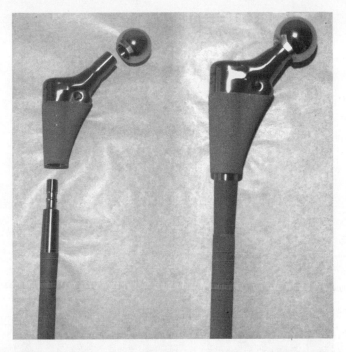

Figure 36   A modular revision prosthesis on left (Zimmer ZMR) consisting of separate head, body, and long stem components. The assembled prosthesis is shown at right.

Courtesy of Zimmer Holdings, Inc.

Modular femoral components are helpful because they give more flexibility in specific anatomic situations. There is, however, an incidence of failure at the junction between the body and the stem in these components.

In unusual circumstances, where an entire section of the bone near the hip is missing, a proximal femoral replacement component may be used. This is sometimes helpful in tumor cases. Larger femoral heads, 36 or 40 mm in diameter, can be used to provide stability in revision cases.

On the acetabular side, larger components may be needed to fill greater defects. A *protrusio shell* can provide

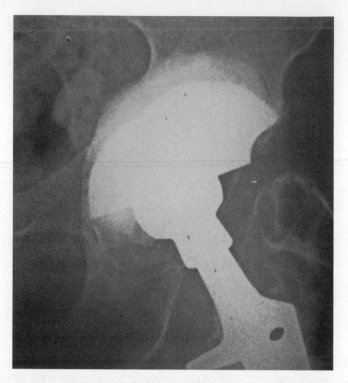

Figure 37 An oblong or specially shaped acetabular component can be used to fill a defect in the bone above the acetabulum.

additional support where there is a defect in the medial or inner portion of the acetabulum. Sometimes a special acetabular *cage* is necessary to bridge a defect in the pelvis or to hold an acetabular component in place if there is no bony support.

An oblong acetabular component may be used when the defect in the socket is wider than normal or has an unusual shape.

Revision components may require supporting fixation such as cables, a straight plate, or a hook shaped trochanteric plate. The supporting fixation may also include a strut of bone taken from a bone bank called an allograft.

If a revision is done for instability, a special *constrained* acetabular component may be used to lock the femoral head into the socket. This is used only after multiple attempts have been made to correct an instability problem. Constrained acetabular components are best used for salvage situations in low demand patients.

In other salvage situations, a bipolar component may be substituted for a total hip replacement because of its wide femoral head and double bearing surfaces.

Recently, an unusual combination of a stem, a bipolar head, and a wide acetabular component has been used to create a *tripolar* arthroplasty. This is felt to be very stable because it has movement and bearing surfaces at three levels.

85. Why is bone grafting sometimes necessary? Where do bone grafts come from?

Bone grafts are sometimes necessary to fill a space where there is a defect in the bone. This is uncommon in primary total hip replacements unless there is an anatomic deformity, but bone grafts are frequently required in a revision setting. A bone graft can be used to reinforce areas where the bone is weak or to restore bone substance where the bone is completely absent.

In revision cases, the bone of the femur is frequently worn away by osteolysis. New bone or additional bone is often required to reinforce the area where the bone has become weak.

Most often the type of bone that is used is called an *allograft*, bone taken from a cadaver donor and then prepared for use in the operating room. Once the bone has been removed, it is tested for any transmissible

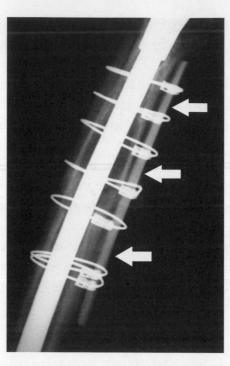

Figure 38   A long stem revision component with a cadaver allograft femoral strut (arrows) on the side. The allograft is fixed with circular cables passed around the bone. It is used to reinforce weakened or osteoporotic bone.

diseases. It is then prepared and freeze-dried. It is sterilized and packaged by a tissue bank for use in the operating room.

Autograft

A bone graft taken from a patient's own body during surgery used to promote healing in another area.

An **autograft** is bone taken from the patient undergoing surgery at the time of the operation. During hip replacement, the bone most often used as a graft is the femoral head which has been dislocated and removed. The femoral head is useful as a graft when it is placed on the lateral side of the acetabulum. Here it can be used to add extra bone to a shallow socket and allow for placement of an acetabular component.

Allografts are used much more than autografts because they can provide a larger amount of bone. Allografts may take the form of femoral cortical struts, morcelized cancellous chips, a femoral head, a tubular segmental graft, or a massive bulk allograft.

Femoral cortical struts are large strips of hard cortical bone which are as wide as one-third to one-half of the circumference of a normal femur. They are placed around the normal cortex of the bone to provide structural reinforcement. They may be used to cover a hole in the bone or to reinforce a thin cortex. If the surgeon has to make a hole, or a window, in the side of the femur to remove cement, the window might be covered with a cortical strut. Cortical struts are held in place by metallic cables placed around the bone.

Small chips of softer morcelized cancellous bone are sometimes packed into the acetabulum to provide reinforcement for the medial wall or to fill a defect within the socket. The chips are inserted and then compacted to fit the defect.

Cancellous chips are also used in the femoral canal for *impaction grafting*. In this procedure, the bone chips are packed inside the femoral canal to provide reinforcement for the bone. The femoral component is then cemented in place.

A femoral head allograft may be used like a femoral head autograft to extend the roof of the acetabulum and provide additional bone for placement of an acetabular component.

In some cases, the entire circumference of a portion of the femur may be weak or absent. A cylindrical tube of bone or *segmental allograft* may then be used. This replaces an entire segment of the proximal femur. The stem of the femoral component is then placed through the segmental allograft and extended into the normal bone below.

In severe cases, where there has been massive bone loss, a *bulk allograft* may be used to substitute for a large portion of the acetabulum or the proximal femur. Bulk allografts are most often needed in hips that have undergone multiple revision procedures or in tumor cases where large amounts of bone must be removed.

Once a graft has been placed, it requires time to incorporate into the normal bone. This process may take several months or longer. It is sometimes helpful to obtain serial x-rays in the months following surgery to determine when the graft has healed. The amount of bone that is incorporated at any one site can be variable and follow up x-rays can be important to determine the structural integrity of the grafted area.

86. Are there greater risks from revision surgery?

Revision surgery is much more extensive than primary total hip replacement and may carry a greater risk of complications.

Revision procedures are often longer and require more anesthesia time. A larger surgical incision and more dissection are required for proper exposure. There tends to be more bleeding and a greater risk of infection due to the extensive amount of tissue dissection.

Nerve complications, such as injuries to the femoral or sciatic nerves, are greater in revision procedures. The nerves are frequently encased in scar and difficult to see.

The need for wider exposure and more retraction in a revision procedure may put added pressure on the nerves.

Since revision cases often involve a deficiency or absence of bone, there is a higher incidence of fixation failure. This is because less bone is available for secure fixation of the components. Dislocation rates in revision procedures are higher than those in primary surgery. In part, this is due to damage to the muscles surrounding the hip joint. Frequently, the muscles are weaker and less likely to maintain the soft tissue tension necessary to keep the hip joint in place.

A leg length discrepancy is also more likely in revisions. This is because the leg may need to be lengthened to make the hip more stable. Beyond this, a large amount of bone loss may make it difficult to accurately judge leg lengths during a revision procedure.

Finally, a larger incision and a greater surgical procedure will tend to be more painful. This makes it more difficult for any patient to become mobile and may lead to a higher incidence of blood clots or postoperative medical problems such as pressure sores or pneumonia.

While some risks such as dislocation can be quantified, others simply reflect the more extensive nature of a revision procedure.

87. Is the rehabilitation after revision surgery longer?

The answer depends upon the extent of the procedure. For most revision surgeries, the rehabilitation is the same as for primary surgery. You will be out of bed on the first or second day after surgery, hospitalized for a short period of time and then move on to a rehabilitation facility.

You will be given antibiotics for the same 24 hours after surgery and will be given anticoagulation to protect against blood clots.

Under some circumstances, however, the normal postoperative rehabilitation has to be modified. If bone grafting is required to maintain the structure of the bone, there might be a longer period of protected weight bearing until the bone heals. Likewise, if extensive bone ingrowth is required to stabilize the prosthesis, then full weight bearing might also be delayed.

Most revision surgeries require a wider surgical exposure than with a primary procedure. This leaves more muscle damage and it may take longer to regain muscle tone and strength. It may be several months before you regain a normal gait. You may need to use an external walking aid such as crutches or a cane for a longer period of time.

All of this depends upon the extent of the procedure and how much healing needs to be done.

As with any orthopaedic procedure it is necessary to make a strong effort at rehabilitation in order to obtain the best possible result.

88. Why do some hip fractures require hip replacement?

Hip replacement either partial (bipolar) or total is sometimes the recommended treatment for an acute fracture.

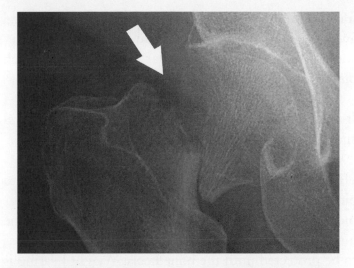

Figure 39   Complete fracture across the neck of the femur (arrow). The head of the femur has broken completely off of the neck and will need replacement.

When a hip fractures across the neck of the femur (subcapital or transcervical fracture) and the fracture is separated or displaced, there is a good chance that the fracture will not heal. Fractures of this type injure the lining or capsule of the hip joint. The blood vessels that supply the femoral head and keep it viable are injured with the capsule. Even if the fracture heals, it may go on to avascular necrosis.

For this reason, hip replacement is often considered the best option for a displaced fracture of the femoral neck. For most acute fractures, bipolar replacement is the treatment of choice. In some circumstances total hip arthroplasty may also be considered.

The surgical approach is similar to the approach for a total hip replacement. An incision may be made from the front (anterior), combined front and side (antero-lateral), from the back (posterior), or combined back and side (posterolateral). The hip joint is exposed, the fractured femoral head removed, the femur is prepared and a femoral stem and head are inserted. The inner and outer bearings of a bipolar component are then placed over the femoral head.

If a total hip arthroplasty is performed, both the femoral and acetabular sides are prepared in the standard manner.

Hip replacement has several advantages compared to pinning or fixation of a fracture. After a hip replacement, patients can bear full weight and walk on the hip joint immediately. After a pinning, the fracture has to be protected until the bone heals. Weight bearing is delayed for several weeks.

Replacement eliminates the risks of the fracture settling and the leg becoming shortened and will prevent rotational deformity of the leg or foot after the fracture has healed. Since the femoral head is replaced, there is no risk of avascular necrosis developing after the fracture has healed.

Hip replacement is a good option for fractures in very osteoporotic bone where the bone is too soft to allow for stable metal fixation.

Hip replacement is a good option for fractures in very osteoporotic bone where the bone is too soft to allow for stable metal fixation. Sometimes replacement is done if a fracture has already undergone pinning but the nail has cut through the soft bone of the femoral head.

Hip replacement may even be considered when a patient simply cannot be partial weight bearing for a prolonged period of time.

Other special circumstances may warrant a hip replacement. If the fracture is caused by a bone tumor (pathologic) and the bone will not heal, it is better to proceed with replacement. Replacement with a long stem is necessary if there are tumor lesions in both the head of the femur and the shaft, which is the long portion of the bone. This protects both of these areas from any further fracture.

Replacement may also be the best choice if there is a fracture of the femoral head where a large portion of the joint surface is involved.

Hip replacement, either bipolar or total, can be used to treat a nonunion of a fracture. This may be a femoral neck fracture, which was previously pinned or an intertrochanteric fracture treated either by a compression screw or an intramedullary hip nail. In older patients, a second attempt to repair the fracture might be difficult and require a bone graft. Hip replacement might be a better second operation. Again this eliminates the need for further healing of the bone.

When hip replacement is done for an intertrochanteric fracture either primary or nonunion, a special larger body prosthesis is sometimes required. The larger body is often a *calcar replacement*.

While hip replacement has advantages compared to pinning, there are some disadvantages and potential risks. The risks are common to any joint replacement. They include dislocation, loosening, groin pain, and infection. Loosening of the fixation is much less an issue for a hip pinning as the hardware can be easily removed.

The original hip replacements were one piece. They were *monoblock* or *unipolar*. In these components, the ball was attached to the stem and inserted as a single piece. A monoblock component may be the best option for an elderly patient who is severely debilitated and will only be moving from his or her bed to a chair. The surgical procedure will be simpler and require less time under anesthesia.

In summary, when a fracture occurs it is always best to try to preserve the patient's own femoral head and hip joint. In fractures where this cannot be done, replacement is the treatment of choice.

89. Is a total hip ever done for fracture instead of a partial or bipolar replacement?

Primary total hip replacement should be considered if there is evidence of osteoarthritis in the joint, which was present before the fracture. This can sometimes be seen on the emergency room x-ray. If the femoral head is deformed or the joint space is narrow, then there is x-ray evidence of osteoarthritis. Sometimes, patients will give a history of having groin and thigh pain or may have already been diagnosed with osteoarthritis. If there is any question of arthritic change involving both sides of the joint, it is best to replace both sides and do a total hip.

The criteria for doing a total rather than a bipolar arthroplasty are not always clear, and sometimes it is a joint decision made between doctor and patient. The metal surface of the bipolar prosthesis pressing against the articular cartilage may cause groin pain similar to the pain of an arthritic hip. This is more likely to occur in a younger more active patient with higher demand. There is some evidence to suggest that for these patients, total hip arthroplasty may provide a longer lasting more pain-free result.

Total hip arthroplasty does, however, have a higher risk of complications such as dislocation than a bipolar replacement.

PART ELEVEN

Other Questions

What can my family do to help?

Can both hips be replaced at the same time?

Can I get pregnant if I have had a total
hip replacement?

More . . .

90. Is hip replacement done for tumors?

For some patients, the answer is yes. Hip replacement can be used to restore function to a hip that is partially destroyed by tumor.

Bone tumors may be either *primary* or *metastatic*. Primary means that the bone itself is the site of origin of the tumor. The tumor has begun growing in that bone and has not spread there from another organ in the body. Metastatic means that the tumor has come from another organ. Its cells will often resemble the original organ and not bone. Hip replacement is most commonly done for metastatic disease. Sometimes the origin of the tumor is known. Other times the metastatic lesion in bone is the first presentation of the tumor. When this happens, a **biopsy** is part of the surgical procedure. Biopsy is removal of a piece of tissue so that it can be examined under a microscope by a tissue specialist called a *pathologist*. The pathologist can identify the type of tumor and tell what organ it came from.

The tumors that most often spread or metastasize to bone are thyroid, breast, lung, kidney, and prostate. Tumors of the blood and bone marrow such as *multiple myeloma* or *leukemia* can also cause pathologic lesions in bone. When a metastatic lesion destroys a large amount of bone, it can cause a *pathologic fracture*. Tumor reconstructions may be difficult because the shape and size of the tumor is always different and the anatomy may vary. There is often a large amount of bleeding during surgery.

The type of operation will depend on the anatomy of the lesion. For primary tumors such as *osteosarcoma* or *chondrosarcoma* the goal of surgery is to remove the entire tumor. A large or *en bloc* resection is carried out.

Biopsy

Removal of a piece of tissue so that it can be examined under a microscope by a pathologist to identify the tissue type and origin.

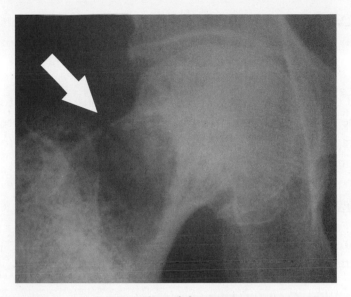

Figure 40 Pathologic fracture (arrow) through abnormal bone in the femoral neck.

When this much bone is removed from the hip, larger specialized components such as a proximal femoral replacement component are sometimes needed. In some cases, a special custom component has to be made to fit the specific anatomy.

In metastatic disease, the goal of surgery is usually to stabilize the fracture rather than to completely remove the tumor. The remaining tumor is treated with radiation or chemotherapy. Again, the type of surgery depends upon the size and location of the tumor. If the tumor is in the femoral head and neck alone, only one side of the joint is replaced. If the tumor involves both the femoral head and the acetabulum, then a total hip replacement is done. When there are metastases that extend to the shaft of the femur, a long stem femoral component is implanted.

Cement fixation is frequently used for the components in tumor cases because the poor quality bone will not support a press fit or bone ingrowth component.

The goals of surgery in metastatic disease are to remove some of the tumor, relieve pain, and promote rapid weight bearing. Surgery is sometimes done to prevent a fracture if the tumor involves a large enough portion of the bone. This is called an *impending pathologic fracture.*

In serious cases, surgery may still be an option to improve a patient's quality of life and to relieve pain.

91. What can my family do to help?

Hip surgery is not just an individual thing. It is a family affair. Even though you are the one having the operation, members of your family can help you get through. They can be there to provide comfort and support, as well as help you with your physical needs before and after surgery.

Your family can help you obtain information about your upcoming operation. (Buying a copy of this book is a good start!) Your family can help you get both written and online information that will help you make an informed decision about hip replacement. If you have elderly parents, aunts, or uncles, it is likely that some of them have friends who have undergone the procedure. They may be able to tell you what to expect from a patient's point of view during your hospital stay and recovery.

It is useful to have a family member go with you to your preoperative consultation at your surgeon's office. There is so much information that it is hard for one person to absorb everything during a single visit. A family member can remember things that you do not and ask questions that you forget to ask. Your spouse may want to ask questions about your needs at home during your postoperative recovery that you would not normally ask.

Family members can also help by donating directed blood. If you have a medical condition that does not allow you to donate your own blood before surgery, then a family member might be able to donate in your place.

Obviously, the most critical time is the day of surgery. It is often soothing and reassuring to have a family member stay with you until you go to the operating room. A family member can also be designated to make medical decisions in the event of a critical emergency.

After surgery, your family can help you with the discharge planning process. If you live alone you may want to stay with a relative for the first few days after your discharge from the hospital or rehabilitation facility. Otherwise, your spouse and immediate family members will need to know what accommodations need to be made at home to assist with your recovery. This may mean rearranging the furniture in your home or putting a bed on the first floor. It may also mean arranging for another family member to stay with you while your spouse goes out to work.

While you are in the hospital or rehabilitation facility, it is good to have a family member who can bring you the little things that you might need, such as an extra pair of pajamas or a pair of slippers.

It is useful to have a family member go with you to your preoperative consultation at your surgeon's office. There is so much information that it is hard for one person to absorb everything during a single visit.

When you get home, your family members will need to help you until you become independent. They can assist with routine activities like bathing, dressing, and preparing meals. In the first few weeks after surgery, you will be unable to drive and it is helpful to have a family member who can take you for your outpatient physical therapy visits.

Most importantly, your family can provide the support and encouragement you need to make a successful recovery.

92. Why do I need antibiotics when I go to the dentist? Do I have to take antibiotics for the rest of my life?

After you have had hip replacement surgery, it is important to make sure that your new hip does not become infected. You want to take steps to prevent bacteria from another part of your body reaching your new hip and causing an infection.

Any injury or procedure that causes bacteria to enter your bloodstream can cause an infection in your hip. An artificial joint is an area that can serve as a focus of infection. There is less blood supply around the components of an artificial joint than there would be to normal tissue. It is harder for the infection fighting cells of your immune system to reach an area around an artificial joint.

You therefore want to protect the joint from any possible source of infection.

Dental work is a common source of *bacteremia*, which is bacteria in the blood. Many different types of bacteria live in the mouth or oral cavity. Your gums are very vascular. That is, they have an extensive blood supply. When the gums bleed, the bacteria in your mouth can enter the bloodstream. If the bacteria reach your artificial joint and grow or colonize, an infection can develop.

For this reason it is necessary to protect your body from *bacteremia* when you are having dental work. Antibiotic protection or *prophylaxis* is recommended. You should have prophylaxis if you are having a procedure such as a root canal, extraction, periodontal or gum surgery, drilling of a cavity or any regular cleaning procedure where there might be bleeding.

If you are not allergic to penicillin, you should take 2 grams of Amoxicillin, Keflex, or Cephradine approximately 1 hour before you go to the dentist. If you cannot take penicillin or are allergic to penicillin, then you should take 600 milligrams of Clindamycin 1 hour before the procedure.

It is generally recommended that patients with hip replacements take prophylactic antibiotics for the rest of their lives. This is especially true for patients at high risk for infection or with a weakened immune system. Patients in this group have conditions which include:

- Rheumatoid arthritis
- Insulin dependent diabetes mellitus
- Transplant recipients
- Collagen vascular diseases such as lupus erythematosus
- Hemophilia
- Leukemia, lymphoma, or other types of cancer
- HIV

In general, you should take antibiotics if you are having any surgical procedure, have an open wound or any major infection in your body.

If you have a question as to whether or not you need antibiotics ask your orthopaedic surgeon.

93. What is minimally invasive surgery?

Minimally invasive surgery is surgery done through a small incision. A surgical incision still has to be made but it is much smaller than a traditional incision. It is thought that a smaller skin incision and more limited surgical approach will result in less dissection and less damage to underlying soft tissues. There will be less cutting of muscle and less disruption of the soft tissue envelope around the hip. This will leave the hip stronger and make rehabilitation faster and easier. Other potential benefits of a minimally invasive procedure are smaller blood loss during surgery, less postoperative pain and more rapid recovery.

The definition of minimally invasive surgery varies by the size of the surgical incision and the type of the surgical approach.

A standard total hip incision is 15–25 cm. The incision for a minimally invasive procedure falls in a range of 6–10 cm for a single incision approach. If a two incision technique is done, then two 3.5–5 cm incisions are made.

The basic operation is still the same. The surgeon does the same bone cutting and drilling as the standard total hip replacement. The femoral head is removed and the acetabulum and femoral canal are reamed and prepared. The same drills, saws, and bone rasps are used for a minimally invasive as for a standard procedure.

The actual femoral and acetabular implants are no different. The sizes and types of components are the same.

What is different is the surgical technique. There are five different approaches to a minimally invasive or small incision technique:

- Anterior single incision
- Anterolateral single incision
- Posterior single incision
- Posterolateral single incision
- Two incisions

Single incision procedures are modifications of a traditional approach. The two incision approach combines a small anterior and a small posterior incision. In this technique, continuous x-ray or fluoroscopy is used to monitor the preparation of the femur and acetabulum as well as the placement of the components. Proponents feel that it does less damage to the main abductor muscles of the hip than other small incision procedures. This means that the hip will be stronger during recovery and afterward.

Not all patients are candidates for minimally invasive surgery. The procedure is best performed on thin, healthy patients with normal anatomy. If there is a complex deformity of the hip, such as a patient who has had DDH, a wider surgical exposure is necessary. Standard incisions are also required in very muscular patients or obese patients with a large body mass index. BMI is the ratio of body weight divided by body height.

Many surgeons feel that small incision procedures allow for faster rehabilitation and a more rapid recovery. It is not clear, however, if the improved recovery times are the result of less invasive surgery. They may be due to a combination of better anesthesia protocols, more aggressive physical therapy and, above all, patient education and motivation.

94. What is computer navigation?

Computer navigation is a new technique in total hip and knee surgery. While it is still under development, it is hoped that computer navigation can help the orthopaedic surgeon be more precise and accurate in his placement of the hip components in the operating room.

Over the years, better instruments have been developed to help the surgeon judge the position of the implant components. While good tools exist, they may not be as precise as a computer.

On the operating table, component position is not always what the surgeon thinks it is or what he would like it to be. This is due to factors such as patient positioning and variable anatomy. Most times the position of components is within an acceptable range and will not affect the success of the operation. Other times there can be a problem. If components are placed at the wrong angle or in the wrong rotation, the joint may be unstable or may not last as long as it should. This would mean the need for an earlier revision procedure.

Computer navigation may help the surgeon determine the orientation of the pelvis or femur. He can get a real time picture of the position of the components before they are permanently inserted.

Some computer systems require a preoperative CT scan to program the patient's anatomy. All navigation systems require tracking devices that are placed on the patient and send signals to the computer in the operating room. Some of the tracking devices simply rest on the patient. Others require drilling of a tracking pin within bone. Sometimes, a small extra incision has to be made to insert the tracking device.

The signals may be sent from the tracking device to the computer either wirelessly or by sterile wires connected to the computer in the room. Initial readings are taken at the start of the procedure so that the computer has a baseline, or reference points, for the patient's individual anatomy. During the procedure, the surgeon monitors the position of his instruments and components on a computer screen within the room. Once he is satisfied, he can proceed with permanent implantation of the components.

Computer navigation is a new technique and is not routinely used in most hospitals for hip replacement. There are several drawbacks. Most computer systems are expensive, and the setup adds extra time to the procedure. Unless the surgeon uses computer navigation on a routine basis, his operating time will be longer. Beyond this, an additional incision is sometimes needed for the tracking device.

Computer navigation is a new technique and is not routinely used in most hospitals for hip replacement.

While initial reports of computer navigation are positive, it is still not known if results are improved enough to justify the extra time, equipment, and expense that the technique requires. Further research is necessary to determine the risks and benefits of computer techniques.

95. What is wrong site surgery? How can it be prevented?

Wrong site surgery is surgery done on the wrong area of the body. In orthopaedic surgery, it usually refers to surgery on the wrong side of the body. That is, surgery is done on the left leg when it is supposed to be done on the right. It can also be surgery which is done on the correct hand or foot but on the wrong finger or toe.

In some areas of the body such as eye, breast, kidney, or brain, wrong sided surgery can be devastating. It can be life threatening or at the very least severely affect the quality of a person's life. In orthopaedic surgery, operating on the wrong arm or wrong leg is not life threatening, but the consequences can still be serious.

Wrong site surgeries are preventable, but they do occur.

JCAHO (The Joint Commission on Accreditation of Healthcare Organizations) has developed a Universal Protocol to address wrong site surgery. It is recommended that before surgery the surgeon confirm the correct side with the patient while the patient is awake. He will then place an indelible ink mark on the operative extremity. The marking should be visible in the operating room.

In the operating room, a "time-out" is performed before the procedure is started. This involves the anesthesiologist, surgeon, nurses, and all other personnel in the operating room. During the time-out, the correct side of surgery is confirmed along with the procedure to be performed, allergies, and other relevant medical information.

If you are having surgery, make sure that your surgeon identifies the correct side with you. You should also remind him of any allergies or skin sensitivities. Use this opportunity to discuss any last minute medical concerns or orthopaedic issues. These might include your post-op medications or the need to correct a pre-operative leg length discrepancy.

96. Can both hips be replaced at the same time?

Many patients have disease in both hips and want to have surgery done on both sides at the same time. Bilateral surgery is an option for healthy patients who are willing to undergo a longer procedure.

Bilateral surgery has several advantages. It means only one hospitalization instead of two. There is only one anesthesia. Rehabilitation is done on both hips at the same time so the total recovery time is not much longer than a single procedure. In other words, you can get it all over with at once.

Not everyone is a candidate for bilateral surgery. It is only done on healthy patients who can tolerate the stress of a bigger procedure. Patients with severe heart disease, lung disease, or other major systemic problem such as diabetes mellitus, immune deficiency, or a blood disorder are not candidates for bilateral surgery. Older, weaker patients should consider doing only one hip at a time. Beyond this, obese patients who will require a wider surgical exposure and have more blood loss are not good candidates. Patients who have a history of blood clots or phlebitis are also at higher risk from bilateral surgery.

From an anatomic standpoint, patients with severe deformity who need complex reconstruction, where time and blood loss are greater than normal, should not consider two hips in one surgery. Examples of this are patients who have had childhood hip disease or previous surgery where a large amount of hardware has to be removed and the surgical approach is difficult.

Besides the prolonged anesthesia, the main risk of surgery is lower postoperative blood count with a greater need for transfusion. Patients who have had bilateral surgery are more likely to need bank blood in the postoperative period. They often need more blood than the two units they can donate for themselves. It is not clear if doing two hips at the same time increases the risk of blood clots and phlebitis as compared to doing two separate procedures. Some studies show that the complication rates for bilateral surgery are a little less than what they would be if two separate procedures were done.

Other benefits from bilateral surgery are less time in the hospital, lower overall cost, and less time off from work.

If the first side in a bilateral procedure takes longer than expected or the blood loss is too great, the surgeon always has the option of stopping after one side and deferring the second procedure until a later date. He may also consider doing two hips in a staged process during the same hospitalization several days apart.

Overall, the percentage of patients who have both hips done as one procedure is small. Nevertheless, bilateral surgery may have some advantage in an active healthy patient who is able to rehabilitate both hips at one time.

97. Can my body be allergic to the total hip components?

Allergy to total hip components is extremely unusual, but it can happen. Part of the problem is that the symptoms of an allergy to metal placed deep within the body differ from a common allergic reaction. If you eat food or take medicine to which you are allergic, you are likely to develop a rash all over your body. You may have swelling, itching, and redness. In extreme cases, you may even get very sick and have trouble breathing. In a metal allergy, the symptoms are a lot less obvious. Very often an allergy to the metal components presents only as local pain within the hip joint or thigh. It may be no different than other causes of a painful total hip. Sometimes there may be redness of the skin or a rash in the area of the implant. While these may be signs of an infection, they may also suggest an allergy to metal.

Unfortunately, there is no simple way to make the diagnosis. Both x-rays and blood tests will be normal. There may not be any local swelling or tenderness. Unless there is a local rash there may be no physical signs at all. Later on, there may be some thinning of the bone, or osteolysis, around the prosthesis but this may take months or even years to develop.

Undoubtedly some allergies to metal are never detected. If the allergy is detected, removal of the components will relieve the pain.

Some patients have skin surface allergy or sensitivity to metals such as nickel. They will typically have a reaction to metals placed in or near the skin such as earrings. A patch test on the skin surface can sometimes detect a surface allergy. The patch test, however, does not correlate well with metal sensitivity within the body.

It is known that patients are more likely to be allergic to cobalt-chromium than titanium. There is no known allergy to the polyethylene, which is used as a liner in most acetabular components.

Cobalt-chromium metal on metal surfaces should probably be avoided in patients with known metal allergies.

If you have had any history that leads you to suspect a metal allergy or sensitivity, inform your orthopaedic surgeon when you are planning your procedure.

98. Can I get pregnant if I have had a total hip replacement?

The answer is yes. Why not? Who is stopping you?

What you really want to know, of course, is if it is safe. Will it damage your hip replacement? Will it have any effect on your baby?

When you can have sex after surgery has been discussed in question 66.

Years ago, hip replacement surgery was almost always done on older people. Pregnancy really wasn't a question. Now as more women are having the operation in their 20s, 30s, and 40s, the question is being asked.

Women can give birth by both normal vaginal delivery and cesarean section after hip replacement surgery. Even though the acetabular component of a hip replacement is placed in the pelvis, it does not affect the normal pelvic anatomy. The size and shape of the pelvis remain the same. There is no effect anatomically on the birth canal. Having a hip replacement does not mean that you will automatically need a cesarean section.

The normal weight gain in pregnancy may place some additional strain on the prosthesis. Some women complain of groin pain on the operated side during the later months of pregnancy. This will usually disappear after the pregnancy is complete.

When you are about to give birth, remind your obstetrician that you have had a hip replacement so that he may be careful in flexing your hip during delivery.

Relatively few studies have been done on pregnancy following total hip replacement. So far, pregnancy has not been shown to have any effect on the long-term survival of the prosthesis. In other words, getting pregnant and having children does not mean that your hip will last for a shorter period of time.

Women in childbearing years are younger and more active. They will place a higher demand on their operated hips and have a longer projected life span. These factors alone outside of pregnancy will most affect the longevity of any prosthetic joint.

If you are considering hip replacement surgery and planning to have a family later on, let your orthopaedic surgeon know. He may want to consider what type of implants he will use for your hip replacement. In particular, the long-term effects of metal on metal surfaces are not yet completely known. Metallic ions have been found within the body though there is no evidence that they affect either the pregnancy or the fetus. Nevertheless, your orthopaedic surgeon may want to discuss the risks and benefits of different bearing surfaces if you are planning to become pregnant later on.

Hip resurfacing is one procedure used in younger patients that has metal on metal joint surfaces.

99. Will my total hip set off an airport metal detector?

If you have had a total hip replacement, you will likely set off the metal detector at an airport security screening facility.

Recent studies show that 90% of all total hip and knee replacements will be detected by a typical walk-through metal detector at an airport.

Recent studies show that 90% of all total hip and knee replacements will be detected by a typical walk-through metal detector at an airport. This type of detector has multiple electrical coils at several levels which can detect metal objects.

Interestingly enough, joint replacements in the upper extremities such as total shoulder or radial head replacements are less likely to set off the alarm. Metal plates and screws are also less likely to create a problem than total hips or total knees.

Studies have shown that titanium and cobalt-chromium metal alloys more commonly trigger an alarm than implants made of stainless steel. Alarms may also be triggered at other types of facilities such as government buildings.

When you are traveling, come to the airport a little earlier to allow extra time for security screening. Advise the TSA security officer before you go through the walk-through detector that you have had a hip replacement. You may also want to present a card given to you by your physician that states that you have had a joint replacement.

The officer will then perform additional screening such as use of a metallic wand or a pat-down.

There is no evidence that the x-ray process itself will have any effect on your joint replacement.

As more and more hip replacements are performed, screening personnel have increased knowledge and ability to screen passengers quickly and effectively in this situation.

If you bring assistive aids such as a cane, crutches, or a walker, they will need to be x-rayed and checked as well.

Remember, always allow extra time when you are going to the airport!

100. Conclusion—Where do I go from here?

Hopefully, the questions and answers in this book have given you something to think about. If you are considering surgery, it is time to review the information and see if there is anything else you need to know.

It is important that you understand how the hip works, what can cause hip problems and what treatment is available. You should know how the procedure is done, how long it will take to recover, and the risks of surgery.

Talk to your friends and family. They can help you with both planning and recovering from surgery. And talk to your orthopaedic surgeon. He has the knowledge and experience you need to make an informed decision.

If you are still looking for more information two organizations to contact are :

American Academy of Orthopaedic Surgeons
Rosemont, Illinois
www.aaos.org

American Association of Hip and Knee Surgeons
Rosemont, Illinois
www.aahks.org

The American Academy of Orthopaedic Surgeons maintains an excellent patient information web site *Your Orthopaedic Connection* (www.orthoinfo.org). YOC has an entire section devoted to joint replacement including articles on:

- Anesthesia for Hip and Knee Surgery
- Joint Revision Surgery—When Do I Need It?
- Preparing for Joint Replacement Surgery
- Total Joint Replacement
- Total Joint Replacement: Questions Patients Should Ask Their Surgeon
- Hip Implants
- Minimally Invasive Total Hip Replacement
- Total Hip Replacement
- Activities After Hip Replacement
- Total Hip Replacement Exercise Guide
- Osteoarthritis of the Hip

YOC also has a computer tutorial on total hip replacement :
www.orthoinfo.org/informedPatient.cfm

Another web site is *Medline Plus* from the National Institutes of Health (NIH) :
www.nlm.nih.gov/medlineplus/hipreplacement.html

It features an interactive tutorial:
www.nlm.nih.gov/medlineplus/tutorials/hipreplacement/htm/index.htm

and a section on Questions and Answers About Hip Replacement from NIH:
www.niams.nih.gov/Health_Info/Hip_Replacement/default.asp

Information about arthritis and related conditions is available from:

The Arthritis Foundation
Atlanta, Georgia
www.arthritis.org

Glossary

A

Acetabulum (Questions 1 and 4): Socket of the hip joint.

Acetabular Labrum (Questions 4, 36, and 43): A ring of fibrocartilage tissue surrounding the hip joint socket.

Acetabular Notch (Question 4): A small recess inside the acetabulum where the ligamentum teres inserts.

Allograft (Questions 68 and 85): Bone that is taken from a cadaver donor and used as a bone graft.

Ankylosing Spondylitis (Question 11): Condition that develops in young men between teenage years and age 40, which causes fusion of joints, particularly in the pelvis and spine.

Antalgic (Questions 14 and 18): A limping gait that avoids pain.

Apparent Leg Length (Questions 18 and 76): A measurement of leg length taken from the umbilicus to the medial malleolus that can be affected by tilting or contraction of the pelvis.

Arthroplasty (Question 6): A procedure performed to reconstruct a diseased or deformed joint. It is commonly used to refer to joint replacement surgery.

Arthroscopic Debridement (Question 36): A shaving or smoothing of a painful arthritic joint surface done through an arthroscope (see also Chondroplasty).

Arthroscopy (Question 36): A surgical technique where surgery on a joint is performed through tiny incisions with a fiberoptic scope, small instruments, and a video camera.

Articular Cartilage (Question 4): The smooth, white tissue that covers the surfaces of a joint. (see also Hyaline Cartilage)

Aspiration (Question 17): A procedure done by needle puncture to remove fluid from a joint.

Autograft (Question 85): A bone graft taken from a patient's own body during surgery used to promote healing in another area.

Avascular Necrosis (AVN) (Question 9): A disease where the blood flow to the femoral head is damaged and bone undergoes necrosis or dies. (see also Osteonecrosis)

B

Bearing Surfaces (Questions 29, 45, and 49): Two surfaces that move against each other in a prosthetic joint.

Biopsy (Question 90): Removal of a piece of tissue so that it can be examined under a microscope by a pathologist to identify the tissue type and origin.

Bipolar (Question 31): A partial hip replacement used to treat fractures and arthritis when the acetabulum is not involved. It consists of a metal stem, a polyethylene inner bearing and a metal outer bearing.

Broach (Question 43): A special orthopaedic chisel used to prepare the medullary canal of the femur. (see also Rasp)

C

Caisson Disease (Question 9): A disease that can cause avascular necrosis. It occurs in deep sea divers who return to the surface too quickly without allowing adequate time to decompress.

Calcar (Question 4): The bone on the inner side of the neck of the femur.

Calcar Replacement (Questions 84 and 88): A special larger body prosthesis that is used to fill the space on the femoral neck if the calcar is worn down or missing.

Capsule (Question 4): The lining tissue that surrounds the hip joint.

Ceramic (Questions 29 and 50): A hard non-metallic material formed by the action of heat and used as a bearing surface in some hip replacements.

Chondroplasty (Question 36): A shaving or smoothing of a painful arthritic joint surface. (see also Arthroscopic Debridement)

Closed Reduction (Questions 30 and 75): A procedure to put a dislocated hip back in place by manipulation.

Cold Weld (Question 46): The metal to metal bond that is formed when the femoral head component is impacted on the Morse taper part of the femoral stem.

Components (Question 1): New parts inserted or implanted in a patient's body. (see also Implants)

Core Decompression (Questions 9 and 20): A surgical procedure to treat avascular necrosis done by drilling the femoral neck and femoral head.

D

Deep Vein Thrombosis (DVT) (Questions 57 and 71): When blood clots form in the deep veins of the leg.

Dislocation: When the ball of the hip joint comes out of the socket.

E

Ectopic Bone (Question 77): Abnormal bone that forms in the soft tissues around a bone or near a joint. (see also Heterotopic Ossification)

Epidural (Question 40): Regional anesthesia given by a small catheter placed outside the lining of the spinal cord.

Extended Trochanteric Osteotomy (Question 83): A technique used in revision surgery where a cut is made in the greater trochanter and femoral shaft to expose the inside of the femoral canal.

F

Femoral Head (Question 4): The round part or ball of the hip joint.

Femoral Neck (Question 4): The section of bone in the hip joint below the femoral head (or ball).

Fovea (Questions 4 and 19): A notch on the surface of the femoral head where blood vessels enter.

Fracture (Question 2): A crack or break in a bone.

G

Gaucher's Disease (Question 11): A metabolic disease that can cause avascular necrosis. Abnormal amounts of fatty material are deposited in different organs of the body.

General Anesthesia (Questions 35 and 40): Anesthesia where a patient is put to sleep and is completely unconscious.

Greater Trochanter (Question 4): Bony prominence located below the femoral neck of the hip where muscles attach that abduct the hip.

H

Hemarthrosis (Question 11): Bleeding into a joint that often occurs with hemophilia.

Hemophilia (Question 11): A disease where absence of a clotting factor in the blood causes abnormal bleeding.

Herniated Nucleus Pulposus (Herniated Disc) (Question 22): A condition where disc material between vertebrae extrudes into the spinal canal causing pressure on nerve roots and leg pain.

Heterotopic Ossification (Question 77): Abnormal bone that forms in the soft tissues around a bone or near a joint. (see also Ectopic Bone)

Hip Arthrodesis (Question 33): Surgical fusion of the ball and socket of the hip joint to form one continuous bone.

Hyaline Cartilage (Question 19): The type of cartilage that covers joint surfaces. (see also Articular Cartilage)

Hybrid Arthroplasty (Question 32): A joint replacement where one component is cemented in place and the other component is press fit.

I

Idiopathic (Question 9): Condition that develops spontaneously with no known cause.

Impaction Grafting (Questions 83 and 85): A procedure where bone chips are packed inside the femoral canal to provide reinforcement for the bone before the prosthesis is inserted.

Implants (Question 1): Prosthetic parts inserted or implanted in a patient's body. (see also Components)

Inferior Vena Cava (Questions 57 and 73): A large vein that carries blood from the lower part of the body to the right side of the heart.

Inner Bearing (Question 31): The inner polyethylene layer of a bipolar prosthesis that sits between the femoral head and the outer bearing metal shell.

Intertrochanteric (Question 4): Area of the femur below the femoral neck between the greater and lesser trochanters.

K

Kyphoplasty (Question 47): A procedure to treat compression fractures in the spine where bone cement is injected into the vertebral body.

L

Leg Length Inequality (Question 76): When one leg is longer or shorter than the other.

Lesser Trochanter (Question 4): Small bony prominence below the femoral neck of the femur where the iliopsoas muscle attaches.

Ligamentum Teres (Question 4): A thick ligament that extends from an area of the acetabulum called the acetabular notch to a point on the femur called the fovea. It carries a portion of the blood supply to the femoral head.

Limited Resurfacing (Question 32): A resurfacing procedure where only the femoral component is applied. This can be done if the hip disease involves only the femoral head and not the acetabulum.

Loose Bodies (Question 36): Free fragments of bone or cartilage within a joint.

Loosening (Questions 21 and 82): When one or both components of a hip replacement is no longer securely fixed to bone.

Lucent Lines (Question 82): Thin, clear lines seen on x-ray between a component and bone or between cement and bone that may indicate component loosening.

M

Mechanical Prophylaxis (Question 57): Mechanical devices such as compression boots used to prevent blood clots.

Metaphysis (Question 43): A wide area of the femur between the femoral neck and shaft of the bone.

Monoblock (Questions 31, 48, and 88): A component that is a single piece with no modular parts. (see also Unipolar)

Monomer (Question 47): A small molecule that may bond chemically to other molecules to form a polymer.

Morse Taper (Question 46): Upper metal portion of the femoral stem component where the head and neck are impacted.

O

One-Stage Exchange Arthroplasty (Question 70): An operation to treat infection where old components are removed and new components are implanted in a single procedure.

Open Reduction (Questions 30 and 75): A procedure to put a dislocated hip back in place by open surgery.

Osteolysis (Question 49): Thinning or loss of bone usually caused by infection or particulate debris.

Osteonecrosis (Question 9): A disease where the blood flow to the femoral head is damaged and bone undergoes necrosis or dies. (see also Avascular Necrosis)

Osteophytes (Questions 6 and 19): Bony prominences that form at the edges of an arthritic joint. (see also Spurs)

Osteotomy (Question 34): An operation where a section of the bone is cut so that the bone may be realigned to a better position.

Outer Bearing (Question 31): The outer metal layer of a bipolar prosthesis that is attached over the inner bearing. The outer bearing makes a joint with the acetabulum.

P

Paget's Disease (Questions 11 and 19): A metabolic disease of bone where bone is rapidly destroyed and then repaired. The rapid rate of bone metabolism causes abnormal appearance and bone deformity.

Pannus (Question 7): Inflamed synovial tissue in a joint with rheumatoid arthritis that invades and destroys joint surfaces.

Partial Hip Replacement (Question 1): A hip joint replacement where only the femur is replaced with an artificial or prosthetic part. The hip joint socket (acetabulum) is left intact.

Particulate Debris (Question 49): Small particles given off in the area of the joint when the polyethylene liner of an acetabular component wears down. It is felt to cause thinning of bone and loosening of components.

Pathologic Fracture (Questions 19 and 90): A fracture which occurs through abnormal bone such as a bone cyst, Paget's disease, or cancer.

Periosteum (Question 77): The outer lining tissue on the surface of bone.

Periprosthetic Fracture (Question 78): A fracture which occurs around or near a prosthetic component.

Polyethylene (Questions 3 and 45): A strong plastic material used as the bearing surface in most acetabular components.

Polymethylmethacrylate (PMMA) (Question 47): Acrylic cement used to hold implants in bone in joint replacement.

Prophylactic Antibiotics (Question 54): Antibiotics given before and after surgery to protect against infection.

Prosthesis: An artificial component or implant used to replace a damaged or diseased body part.

Pulmonary Embolus (Question 71): A blood clot in the lung.

R

Rasp (Question 43): A special orthopaedic chisel used to prepare the medullary canal of the femur. (see also Broach)

Reduction (Question 74): A procedure to put a dislocated hip back in place either by manipulation or open surgery.

Regional Anesthesia (Question 40): Anesthesia where a patient is awake but the lower part of the body is numb and the patient cannot feel any pain.

Resurfacing (Question 32): A type of hip replacement that preserves the femoral neck and inner portion of the femoral head. Only the articular cartilage and outer portion of the femoral head are removed.

Revision (Question 81): A second surgical procedure that is done to replace one or more parts of the original hip replacement.

S

Sclerotic (Questions 6 and 19): Hard dense bone that forms beneath the surface in an arthritic joint.

Septic Arthritis (Question 20): Infection in a joint.

Shaft (Questions 3 and 4): The long portion of a bone. In the femur it is the segment between the hip and the knee.

Sickle Cell Anemia (Question 11): A disease found predominantly in African Americans or people of African descent. Round red blood cells take on a crescent or sickle shape and cannot pass through small vessels in the body. This can cause avascular necrosis in the hip.

Spinal (Question 40): Regional anesthesia given by a single injection placed inside the lining that surrounds the spinal cord.

Spurs (Question 6): Bony prominences that form at the edges of an arthritic joint. (see also Osteophytes)

Stasis (Question 71): When blood sits or pools in a vein and does not flow normally.

Subtrochanteric: Part of the femur below the two trochanters.

Superior Vena Cava (Question 69): A large vein in the chest that brings blood from the head, neck, arms, and chest back to the heart.

Synovial Chondromatosis (Question 36): A condition where multiple loose bodies form in the joint from articular cartilage.

Synovium (Questions 4 and 7): Lining tissue inside a joint which secretes synovial fluid to lubricate and nourish the joint.

T

Template (Questions 19 and 76): A tracing or outline of different sized hip components placed over an x-ray before surgery to estimate the size and position of the implants in a hip replacement.

Trabecular (Question 19): A cross-hatched pattern seen on an x-ray in the bone of the femoral head and femoral neck.

Thrombocytopenia (Question 57): A condition where there is a low platelet count in blood.

Total Hip Replacement (Question 1): A hip joint replacement where both the ball of the hip joint (femoral head) and the hip joint socket (acetabulum) are removed and replaced with artificial or prosthetic parts.

Trial Reduction (Question 43): Part of a hip replacement procedure where trial components are inserted and the femoral head is placed in the socket. The joint is then checked for alignment and stability before permanent components are inserted.

Trochanteric Osteotomy (Question 75): A technique where the greater trochanter is detached from the femur and re-attached lower down to tighten muscles and create greater stability.

True Leg Length (Questions 18 and 76): A measurement of the length of leg without regard to tilting or deformity of the pelvis. The measurement is taken from a point on the front of the pelvis called the anterior superior iliac spine to the medial malleolus.

Two-Stage Exchange Arthroplasty (Question 70): Treatment for total hip infections where components are removed in a first procedure and new components are reimplanted several weeks later when the infection has cleared.

U

Unipolar (Questions 31 and 88): A component that is a single piece with no modular parts. (see also Monoblock)

Index

abduction pillow, 105, 176
abduction slides, 145
acetabular cage, 202
acetabular labrum, tear of, 85
acetabular notch, 11
acetabulum, 2, 3, 10
acetaminophen, 56, 128
acetylsalicylic acid. *See* nonsteroidal anti-
inflammatory drugs
acrylic cement, 112
activities of daily living (ADL), physical
therapy and, 144
activity; *See also* exercises
arthritis and, 52
addiction, pain medication and, 128
ADL. *See* activities of daily living
airport metal detector, total hip
replacement and, 230–231
alcoholism, dislocations and, 171
alkaline phosphatase test, for heterotopic
ossification, 183
allergy. *See* hypersensitivity reaction
allografts, 157, 203–205
bulk, 206
segmental, 205–206
alumina, 122
American Academy of Orthopaedic
Surgeons, 231
deep vein thrombosis prophylaxis
and, 136
American Association of Hip and Knee
Surgeons, 232
American College of Chest Physicians,
deep vein thrombosis prophylaxis
and, 137
American College of Rheumatology,
17
amoxicillin, 219
Ancef. *See* cefazolin

Andry, Nicholas, 98
anemia, total hip replacement and,
187
anesthesia
catheter and, 132
epidural, 97–98, 127
general, 83, 95–98, 127
local, 127
regional, 95–98
spinal, 97–98
for total hip replacement, 95–98
anesthesiologist, 96
ankle pumps, 144
ankylosing spondylitis, 13
arthritis and, 27
antalgic gait, 32
antibiotics
dental visits and, 218–220
prophylactic, 130, 219
total hip replacement and, 130–131,
159–162
broad spectrum, 160
injections, 161
intravenous, 160
peripherally inserted central catheter
for, 160–161
sensitivity test and, 160
anticoagulation. *See* blood thinners
apparent leg length, 38, 177
Arixtra. *See* fondaparinux
arterial insufficiency, 49
arthritis, 12, 13
activity and, 52
bending and, 32–33
cane use and, 54
causes of, 26–28
childhood disease, secondary to, 13
in children, 23–26
crepitus and, 34

arthritis (*continued*)
diagnosis of, 36–37
aspiration, 37
blood tests, 37
family history, 36
medical history, 36
MRI, 37, 44–46
physical examination, 36–42
x-ray, 37, 42–44
disc herniation *vs.*, 48
exercise and, 52
flexion contracture and, 32, 33
juvenile, 16
NSAIDs for, 55–57
pain and
causes of, 30–31
duration of, 30–31
limping and, 31–32
location of, 30
post-traumatic, 13, 18–19
dislocation and, 19
fracture and, 18–19
total hip replacement after, 67
rheumatoid, 13, 16–18
diagnosis of, 17
incidence of, 16
rotational deformity and, 32
septic, MRI and, 45
shoe tying and, 32–33
short leg and, 31–32
spinal stenosis and, 48
weight loss and, 52–53
Arthritis Foundation, 233
arthrogram, 47
component loosening and, 47, 195
arthroplasty
bipolar. *See* bipolar hip replacement
hybrid, 73
for osteoarthritis, 16
arthroscopic debridement, 86
arthroscopy, 84–87
for bone spurs, 85
complications of, 86
future of, 87
for osteoarthritis, 16, 85–86
for osteophytes, 85
procedure, 84
articular cartilage, 11, 12, 14
aspiration, infection and, 158, 161
aspirin. *See* nonsteroidal anti-inflammatory
drugs
assistive aids, 137–138, 145–147
bath bench, 147
commode, 147

after hip replacement, 137–138
leg lifter, 145
long handle sponge, 146
long shoe horn, 146
raised toilet seat, 147
reacher/grabber, 146, 147
scratcher, 146
shower chair, 147
sock donner, 145, 146
Austin Moore prosthesis, 6, 69, 111
autograft, 204
autologous blood donation, 94, 132
avascular necrosis (AVN), 13, 20–23
causes of, 20–22
core decompression of, 23, 82–84
diagnosis of, 22–23
idiopathic, 22
MRI and, 45
symptoms of, 20, 22
total hip replacement after, 67
treatment of, 22–23
AVN. *See* avascular necrosis

bacteremia, 218–219
bacteria, infections and, 159–162
Bateman, James, 69
bath bench, 147
bearing surfaces, 62, 106, 108, 119
bed, exercises in, 144–145
Benadryl, for hypersensitivity reaction, 187
bending, arthritis and, 32–33
bilateral hip replacement, 224–225
bipolar arthroplasty. *See* bipolar hip
replacement
bipolar hip replacement, 68–73, 209–210
anatomy of, 70–71
risks of, 73
total hip replacement *vs.*, 212
x-ray of, 72
bipolar prosthesis. *See* bipolar hip replacement
bladder scan, 133
blood clot; *See also* deep vein thrombosis
pulmonary embolism and, 136
after total hip replacement, 129
blood donation
autologous, 94, 132
before total hip replacement, 94–95
blood loss during surgery, blood transfusion
for, 131
blood thinners, 133–137
aspirin, 135–136
compression stockings and, 133
Coumadin, 134, 136, 167, 169

Index

dalteparin (Fragmin), 135, 136
enoxaparin (Lovenox), 135, 136
fondaparinux (Arixtra), 135, 136
heparin (low molecular weight),
    134–135, 136, 167, 169
pneumatic compression devices and, 133
Warfarin, 134, 167
blood transfusion, 131–132; See also blood
    donation
    directed, 132, 217
board certified, 100
bone cement, 112–115
bone grafts, 203–206
    for avascular necrosis, 23
bone scan
    component loosening and, 196
    infection and, 158
bone spurs
    arthroscopy for, 85
    on x-ray, 44
bone tumors
    biopsy of, 214
    chondrosarcoma, 214–215
    en bloc resection of, 214–215
    hip replacement for, 5, 215–216
    impending pathologic fracture and,
        216
    metastatic, 214, 215, 216
    osteosarcoma, 214–215
    pathologic fracture and, 44, 214, 215
    primary, 214
    on x-ray, 44
bone-on-bone, on x-ray, 14, 15, 43
broach, 103
broad spectrum antibiotics, 160
bulk allograft, 206

caisson disease, 21
calcar, 11
    replacement, 200, 211
cancellous chips, 205
cane, use of, 54
    arthritis and, 52–53
    after total hip replacement, 138
capsule, 11
case manager, 143
catheter, urinary, 132–133, 188
cefazolin, 130, 160
celecoxib (Celebrex), 57
cement
    acrylic, 112
    antibiotic loaded, 163
    removal of, 198–199
cement spacer, 163

Cephradine, 219
ceramics, 62, 109, 121–123
certified registered nurse anesthetist
    (CRNA), 96
Charnley, Sir John, 6, 112–113
childhood disease, arthritis secondary to, 13
children, arthritis in, 23–26
Chondroitin, 57–59
chondroplasty, 86
chondrosarcoma, 214–215
circulating nurse, 101
Clindamycin, 130, 160, 219
closed reduction, 64, 173–174, 176
cobalt-chromium components, 107–108
    hypersensitivity reaction to, 227–228
cold weld, 112
commode, 147
components
    bearing surfaces, 106, 108
    bone cement and, 112–115
    breaking of, 190–191
    ceramics, 109
    cobalt-chromium, 107–108
    composition of, 106–109
    failure of, 190–191
    hypersensitivity reaction to, 226–228
    implantation of, 110–112
    loosening of, 190, 192–197
    metal on metal, 109
    modular, 115–119
    polyethylene, 6, 108, 109
    porous surfaces of, 107, 111, 112
    titanium, 107, 109
compression stockings, 133
computed tomography (CT) scan
    pus/fluid collection on, 158
    spiral, for pulmonary embolism, 168
computer navigation, hip replacement and,
    222–223
congenital shortening, 39
constrained acetabular compartment,
    175, 203
core decompression, 45
    for avascular necrosis, 23, 82–84
    procedure, 83
cortisone injections, 59–60
Coumadin, 134, 136, 167, 169
cracking noise. See crepitus
C-reactive protein, infection and, 157,
    161
creeping substitution, 22
crepitus, 34
CRNA. See certified registered nurse
    anesthetist

crutches, as assistive aid, 137–138
CT scan. *See* computed tomography scan
cup arthroplasty, 6
cysts, subchondral, 14

daily activities, 32–33
dalteparin, 135, 136
DDH. *See* developmental dysplasia of hip
deep vein thrombosis (DVT), 133
   Doppler study for, 165
   incidence of, 164
   inferior vena cava filter for, 167
   MRI and, 166
   post-thrombotic syndrome and,
      166
   prophylaxis; *See also* blood thinners
      American Academy of Orthopaedic
         Surgeons clinical guidelines for,
         136
      American College of Chest Physicians
         recommendation for, 137
   risk factors for, 164
   symptoms of, 165
   treatment of, 166–167
   ultrasound for, 165
   venography for, 165
deformities, on x-ray, 43
dentist, antibiotics and, 218–220
Department of Health and Human
      Services National Hospital
      Discharge Survey, 7
developmental dysplasia of hip (DDH),
      23–26
   total hip replacement after, 64
diclofenac (Voltaren), 57
dietary supplements, 58
diflunisal (Dolobid), 57
Dilaudid. *See* hydromorphone
Diplomate of the American Board of
      Orthopaedic Surgery, 100
directed blood transfusion, 132, 217
disc herniation, 47–48
   arthritis *vs.*, 48
dislocation brace, 176
dislocations, 169–173
   alcoholism and, 171
   avascular necrosis and, 21
   incidence of, 169–170
   post-traumatic arthritis and, 19
   prevention of, 139–141, 144, 151
   reasons for, 171–172
   reduction procedure for, 173–176
   resurfacing and, 75
distended bladder, 133

Doppler study, deep vein thrombosis and,
      165
driving, after total hip replacement, 148,
      149–150
dysbaric disease, 21

ectopic bone. *See* heterotopic ossification
elective surgery, 5
en block resection, of bone tumor,
      214–215
endotracheal (ET) tube, 97
enoxaparin, 135, 136
enteric-coated aspirin (Ecotrin), 57
Enterococcus, 160
epidural anesthesia, 97–98, 127
erythrocyte sedimentation rate (ESR), 17
   infection and, 157, 161
ESR. *See* erythrocyte sedimentation rate
ET tube. *See* endotracheal tube
etodolac (Lodine), 57
exercises
   arthritis and, 52
   for hip strengthening, 144–145
      in bed, 144–145
      sitting, 145
      standing, 145
   physical therapy and, 143–144
extended trochanteric osteotomy, 199

family support, 216–218
Farrar, 120
Fellow of the American Academy of
      Orthopaedic Surgeons, 100
femoral cortical struts, 205
femoral head, 2, 3, 10
   necrosis of, 20
   sizes of, 117
femoral neck, 10
femoral stems, 117, 118
fever, total hip replacement and, 187
fibrocartilage, 11
fixation, hip replacement *vs.*, 210
flexion contracture, 32, 33, 39–40, 176
fluoroscopy, 174
fondaparinux, 135, 136
four prong cane, 138
fovea, 11
fractures
   avascular necrosis and, 21
   hip replacement for, 5, 208–212
      advantages of, 210–211
      disadvantages of, 211
      fixation *vs.*, 210
      location of, 209

pinning *vs.*, 210
total *vs.* partial/bipolar, 212
intraoperative, 184–185
incidence of, 184
treatment of, 184–185
MRI and, 45
periprosthetic, 185
post-traumatic arthritis and, 18–19
Fragmin. *See* dalteparin
full arc knee extensions, 145
fusion, for osteoarthritis, 16

gadolinium, in MRI/MRI venography, 166
gait evaluation, 41
gastrointestinal complications, after surgery,
188
Gaucher's disease, 13
arthritis and, 27
general anesthesia, 83, 95–98, 127
genitourinary complications, after surgery,
188
Gentamycin, 163
Glucosamine, 57–59
gluteal sets, 144
gram-negative bacteria, 160
gram-positive bacteria, 160
greater trochanter, 11
group D Streptococcus, 160
gynecologic disease, pain and, 49

handicap parking, 150
heel slides, 144
hemarthrosis, 27
hematocrit, low, blood transfusion
for, 131
hemoglobinopathies, 21
hemophilia, 13
arthritis and, 27
hemoptysis, 168
heparin, low molecular weight, 134–135,
136, 167, 169
hernia, inguinal, 49
herniated nucleus pulposus, 47–48
heterotopic ossification (H.O.),
180–184
causes of, 180
radiation for, 183
risk groups of, 182–183
surgery for, 183, 184
symptoms of, 181–182
treatment of, 182
x-ray of, 181
hip abduction, 145
hip arthrodesis, 78

hip extension, 145
hip fusion, 77–81
history of, 79
pain and, 78
procedure, 79
risks of, 80
spica cast and, 80
total hip replacement after, 66, 81
x-ray of, 78
hip joint
anatomy of, 10–12
acetabular notch, 11
acetabulum, 2, 3, 10
articular cartilage, 11, 12, 14
calcar, 11
capsule, 11
femoral head, 2, 3, 10
femoral neck, 10
fibrocartilage, 11
fovea, 11
greater trochanter, 11
intertrochanteric, 11
labrum, 11
lesser trochanter, 11
ligamentum teres, 11
shaft, 11
subtrochanteric, 11
synovium, 11
arthritis and, 12, 13
degeneration of, 12
disease of, 12–13
hip joint ball. *See* femoral head
hip joint socket. *See* acetabulum
hip replacement
assistive aid after, 137–138, 145–147
bilateral, 224–225
bipolar, 68–73; *See also* bipolar hip
replacement
bone tumors and. *See* bone tumors
ceramic on ceramic, 121–123
components of, 2
computer navigation, 222–223
elective surgery and, 5
fracture and. *See* fractures
implants and, 2
long-term results of, 63
metal on metal, 109, 119–121
minimally invasive surgery for, 220–222
incisions in, 220–221
monoblock, 68, 116, 211
partial, 2, 3, 6; *See also* bipolar hip
replacement
population and, 62–63
procedure, 101–105

hip replacement (*continued*)
  abduction pillow after, 105
  incision closure, 104
  incision dressing, 104–105
  initial incision, 101–102
  irrigation, 104
  patient position, 101
  trial reduction, 104
  revision surgery and. *See* revision
    procedure
  total. *See* total hip replacement
  unipolar, 68, 211
  weight and, 52–53
  wrong site surgery and, 223–224
hip strengthening, exercises for, 144–145
  in bed, 144–145
  sitting, 145
  standing, 145
HLA-B27, 27
H.O. *See* heterotopic ossification
Homan's sign, 165
home precautions, after total hip
    replacement, 140
hyaline cartilage, 43
hybrid arthroplasty, 73
hybrid replacement, 112
hydromorphone, 128
hypersensitivity reaction
  Benadryl for, 187
  to cobalt-chromium, 227–228
  to components, 226–228
  to medications, 187–188
  metal and, 121, 227–228
  to nickel, 227
  patch test and, 227
  sensitivity test and, 160
  to titanium, 227
hypotension, anemia and, 187

ibuprofen (Motrin, Advil), 57, 128
ilium, 10
image intensifier, 83
impaction grafting, 199, 205
implant manufacturer representative, 101
implants, 2
Indium scan
  component loosening and, 196
  infection and, 158
indomethacin (Indocin), 57, 182, 183
infection, 13
  antibiotics and, 130–131
  arthritis and, 26
  arthrogram for, 47
  sources of, 161

superficial, 159
surgery for, 162–163
total hip replacement and, 67–68,
    156–159
  antibiotics and, 159–162
  aspiration and, 158
  diagnosis of, 157
  incidence of, 156
  laboratory tests and, 157
  risk factors of, 157
  symptoms of, 157
  treatment of, 159–162
  wound debridement, 159
  x-rays and, 158
infectious disease specialist, 160, 161
inferior vena cava filter, 136–137
  for deep vein thrombosis, 167
inguinal hernia, 49
injections, of antibiotics, 161
inner bearing, 70
INR. *See* International Normalized Ratio
insurance coverage, 143
International Normalized Ratio (INR),
    Coumadin and, 134
intertrochanteric, 11
intravenous (IV) medication, 127–128
  antibiotics, 160
ions, 121
ischium, 10
IV. *See* intravenous medication

Jackson, Bo, 153
JCAHO. *See* Joint Commission on
    Accreditation of Healthcare
    Organizations
Joint Commission on Accreditation of
    Healthcare Organizations
    (JCAHO), wrong site surgery and,
    224
juvenile arthritis, 16

Keflex, 219
ketoprofen (Orudis), 57
ketorolac (Toradol), 57
knee raises, 145
kyphoplasty, 115

labrum, 11, 103
laryngeal mask airway (LMA), 97
lateral decubitus position, in arthroscopy,
    84
leg length discrepancy, 39
leg length inequality, 176–180
leg lifter, 145

lesser trochanter, 11
ligamentum teres, 11
limited resurfacing, 77
limping, pain and, 31–32
LMA. *See* laryngeal mask airway
local anesthesia, 127
long handle sponge, 146
long shoe horn, 146
loose bodies, 85
loosening, in hip replacement, 190, 192–197
    diagnosis of, 192, 194
        bone scan, 196
        Indium scan, 196
        x-ray, 192, 193, 194, 195, 196
    physical examination, 193
    symptoms of, 192
Lovenox. *See* enoxaparin
low friction arthroplasty, 6
low molecular weight heparin, 134–135, 136
lucent lines, 192, 194
lysis, infection and, 158

magnetic resonance arthrogram (MR arthrogram), 47
magnetic resonance imaging (MRI), 37, 44–46
    arthrogram and, 47
    avascular necrosis and, 45
    contraindications of, 46
    deep vein thrombosis and, 166
    fractures and, 45
    septic arthritis and, 46
    transient osteoporosis, 45–46
    tumors and, 46
McKee, 120
mechanical prophylaxis, 133
medication for pain. *See* pain medication
Medline Plus, 232–233
meloxicam (Mobic), 57
mesenchymal cells, 180–181
metal detector, total hip replacement and, 230–231
metal on metal components, 109, 119–121
    hypersensitivity reaction to, 121, 227–228
metaphysis, 103
metastatic bone tumor, 214, 215, 216
methicillin-resistant Staph aureus (MRSA), 160
mobility, limited, 4
modular components, 115–119, 172, 201
monoblock hip replacement, 68, 116, 211
monomers, 113

Moore, Austin, 6, 68–69
morphine, 127, 128
Morse taper, 112
MR arthrogram. *See* magnetic resonance arthrogram
MRI. *See* magnetic resonance imaging
MRSA. *See* methicillin-resistant Staph aureus
muscle atrophy, 38

nabumetone (Relafen), 57
naproxen (Aleve, Naprosyn), 57
National Institutes of Health (NIH), 232–233
necrosis, 20
nerves, injury to, 185–187
    causes of, 186
    surgery for, 186
    symptoms of, 186
neuropathy, pain and, 49
nickel, hypersensitivity reaction to, 227
NIH. *See* National Institutes of Health
nonsteroidal anti-inflammatory drugs (NSAIDs), 55–57, 128, 135–136
    arthritis and, 52–53
    contraindications of, 56
    for heterotopic ossification, 182, 183
    mechanism of action, 55
    side effects of, 56
NSAIDs. *See* nonsteroidal anti-inflammatory drugs
nutritional supplements, 58

oblong acetabular component, 202
occupational therapist, 144
one-stage exchange arthroplasty, 163
open reduction, 64, 174, 176
operating room, 96–97
    medical personnel in, 100–101
    time-out procedure in, 224
oral medication
    for blood thinners, 133
    for pain, 127–128
Orthopaedia or the Art of Correcting and Preventing Deformities in Children, 98
orthopaedic surgeon, 98–100
    board certified, 100
    education of, 99
    residency and, 99
osteoarthritis, 5, 13
    arthroplasty for, 16
    arthroscopy for, 16, 85–86
    definition of, 13

osteoarthritis (*continued*)
  fusion for, 16
  incidence of, 13–14
  osteotomy for, 16
  pain and, 15–16
  resurfacing for, 16
  symptoms of, 14
  total hip replacement for, 16
  triggers of, 14
osteoblasts, 181
osteocytes, 181
osteolysis, 120
osteomyelitis, 26
osteonecrosis, 20–23; *See also* avascular
      necrosis
osteopathic physician, 100
osteophytes, 14, 44
  arthroscopy for, 85
osteoporosis, 16
  MRI and, 45
osteosarcoma, 214–215
osteotomy, 65, 81–82
  for avascular necrosis, 23
  extended trochanteric, 199
  for osteoarthritis, 16
  reconstructive, total hip replacement
      after, 66
  trochanteric, 175
outer bearing, 70
oxaprozin (Daypro), 57

PA. *See* physician's assistant
PACU. *See* post anesthesia care unit
Paget's disease, 13
  arthritis and, 28
  on x-ray, 44
pain
  arterial insufficiency and, 49
  avascular necrosis and, 22
  disc herniation and, 47–48
  gynecologic disease and, 49
  herniated nucleus pulposos and, 47–48
  hip fusion and, 78
  hip replacement and, 4–5
  inguinal hernia and, 49
  neuropathy and, 49
  osteoarthritis and, 15–16
  spinal stenosis and, 48
  urologic problems and, 49
pain medication
  addition to, 128
  catheter and, 132
  intravenous, 127–128
  oral, 127–128

patient controlled analgesia, 127–128
  per os, 128
  total hip replacement and, 127–128
pannus, 17
paralytic ileus, 188
partial hip replacement, 2–3; *See also* bipolar
      hip replacement
  history of, 6
particulate debris, 120
patch test, hypersensitivity reaction and, 227
pathologic fracture
  bone tumor and, 44, 214, 215
  impending, 216
patient controlled analgesia (PCA),
      127–128
PCA. *See* patient controlled analgesia
pelvic obliquity, 178
pelvic osteotomy, 82
pelvic tilt, 178
penicillin, 130, 219
Percocet, 128
periosteum, 180
peripheral neurologic examination, 41
peripheral neuropathy, 32
peripherally inserted central catheter
      (PICC line), for antibiotics, 160
Perthes disease, 23–26
  total hip replacement after, 66
phlebitis, 164
physiatrist, 142
physical examination, 36–42
  apparent leg length, 38
  congenital shortening, 39
  flexion contracture, 39–40
  gait evaluation, 41
  leg length discrepancy, 39
  muscle atrophy, 38
  peripheral neurologic examination, 41
  range of abduction, 40
  range of adduction, 40
  range of motion, 40
  range of rotation, 40
  Thomas test, 39
  tilted pelvis and, 38
  Trendelenburg test, 41
  true leg length, 38–39
physical therapy, 137, 142, 143–144
  after total hip replacement, 129
physician's assistant (PA), 100
PICC line. *See* peripherally inserted central
      catheter
pinning, hip replacement *vs.*, 210
piroxicam (Feldene), 57
platelets, low. *See* thrombocytopenia

PMMA. *See* polymethylmethacrylate
pneumatic compression devices, 133
P.O. (per os) medication, 128; *See also* oral
    medication
polio, 32
polyethylene, 6, 108, 109
polymerization, 113
polymethylmethacrylate (PMMA), 113
porous surfaces, of components, 107,
    111, 112
post anesthesia care unit (PACU), 98
post-thrombotic syndrome, deep vein
    thrombosis and, 166
post-traumatic arthritis, 13, 18–19
    dislocation and, 19
    fracture and, 18–19
    total hip replacement after, 67
pregnancy, total hip replacement and,
    228–229
primary bone tumor, 214
prophylactic antibiotics, 130, 219
prostate, enlargement of, catheter for, 132
prosthesis, 6
    bipolar. *See* bipolar hip replacement
protamine sulfate, for low molecular weight
    heparin, 135
protrusio, on x-ray, 44
protrusio shell, 201–202
pubis, 10
pulmonary embolism, 136, 165, 167–169
    diagnosis of, 168
    spiral CT scan for, 168
    symptoms of, 168
    treatment of, 169
pulse oximeter, 168
pus/fluid collection, infection and, 158

quad cane, 54, 138

radiation therapy
    avascular necrosis and, 21
    heterotopic ossification and, 183
raised toilet seat, 147
range of abduction, 40
range of adduction, 40
range of motion, 40
range of rotation, 40
rasp, 103
reacher/grabber, 146, 147
reconstructive osteotomy, total hip replace-
    ment after, 66
reduction procedure, for dislocations,
    173–176
regional anesthesia, 95–98

registered nurse first assistant (RNFA), 100
rehabilitation
    after revision procedure, 207–208
    after total hip replacement, 126, 141–143
reinfusion drain, 131
residency, orthopaedic surgeon and, 99
resurfacing, 62, 73–77
    advantages of, 75
    for avascular necrosis, 23
    components of, 73, 74
    contraindications of, 76
    dislocations and, 75
    limited, 77
    for osteoarthritis, 16
    procedure, 75–76
    revision of, 77
    success rate of, 76–77
retractors, 186
revision procedure, 4
    rehabilitation after, 207–208
    risks from, 206–207
    of total hip replacement, 190–192,
        197–200
revision surgery, 4
rheumatoid arthritis, 13, 16–18
    diagnosis of, 17
    incidence of, 16
rheumatoid factor, 17
RNFA. *See* registered nurse first assistant
rotational deformity, 32

scar tissue, 197
SCFE. *See* slipped capital femoral epiphysis
sclerotic, 14, 43
scratcher, 146
scrub nurse, 101
segmental allograft, 205–206
sensitivity test, antibiotics, 160
septic arthritis, MRI and, 45
sex, after total hip replacement, 150–151
shaft, 6
shoe lift, 179
shoe tying, arthritis and, 32–33
short arc knee extensions, 145
short leg, 31–32
shower chair, 147
sickle cell anemia, 13
    arthritis and, 27–28
sitting exercises, 145
slipped capital femoral epiphysis (SCFE),
    23–26
    total hip replacement after, 65
Smith-Petersen, Marius, 6
social worker, 143

sock donner, 145, 146
spinal anesthesia, 97–98
spinal stenosis, 48
    arthritis and, 48
sport activities, after total hip replacement,
        152–153
spurs, 14
standing block test, 178
standing exercises, 145
Staph aureus, 160
Staph epidermidis, 160
stasis, 164
steroid injections, 59–60
steroid therapy, avascular necrosis and, 22
straight cane, 54, 138
straight catheterization, 133
straight leg raises, 144
subchondral bone, sclerosis of, 14
subchondral cysts, 14
subcutaneous injection, blood thinners and,
        133, 135
subtrochanteric, 11
sulindac (Clinoril), 57
superficial infection, 159
superior vena cava, PICC line and, 161
swimming, 152
synovial chondromatosis, 85
synovium, 11, 17

template, x-ray as, 44
tenosynovitis, 17
Thomas test, 39
thrombocytopenia, low molecular weight
        heparin and, 135
tilted pelvis, 38
time-out procedure, 224
titanium components, 107, 109
    hypersensitivity reaction to, 227–228
Tobramycin, 163
tolmetin (Tolectin), 57
total hip replacement, 2–3
    airport metal detector and, 230–231
    anesthesia for, 95–98
    antibiotics and, 130–131, 159–162
        broad spectrum, 160
        injections, 161
        intravenous, 160
        peripherally inserted central catheter
            for, 160–161
        sensitivity test and, 160
    after avascular necrosis, 67
    blood clot after, 129
    blood donation before, 94–95
    cane, use of, 138

after developmental dysplasia of hip, 64
dislocation precautions after, 139–141,
        144, 151
driving and, 148, 149–150
after hip fusion, 66, 81
history of, 6
home precautions after, 140
hospital stay after, 141
after infection, 67–68
infection and, 67–68, 156–159
    antibiotics and, 159–162
    aspiration and, 158
    diagnosis of, 157
    incidence of, 156
    laboratory tests and, 157
    risk factors of, 157
    symptoms of, 157
    treatment of, 159–162
    wound debridement, 159
    x-rays and, 158
long-term failure of, 153
medical clearance for, 92
medical complications from, 187–188
mobilization after, 128–130
nerve injury during, 185–187
orthopaedic surgeon and, 98–100
for osteoarthritis, 16
pain medication and, 127–128
partial/bipolar hip replacement vs., 212
after Perthes disease, 66
physical therapy after, 129
postoperative, 126
postoperative pain, 127–128
after post-traumatic arthritis, 67
pregnancy and, 228–229
preoperative, 90–94
preparation for, 90–94
previous hip surgery and, 63–68
rehabilitation after, 126, 141–143
revision procedure of, 190–192, 197–200
    custom components in, 200–203
sex after, 150–151
after slipped capital femoral epiphysis,
        65
sport activities after, 152–153
vessels injury during, 185–187
weight bearing after, 129, 137–138
working after, 148–149
wound care after, 141
trabecular pattern, on x-ray, 43
transient osteoporosis, MRI and, 45
transplants, avascular necrosis and, 22
Trendelenburg gait, 32
Trendelenburg test, 41

trial reduction, 104
tripolar arthroplasty, 203
trochanteric osteotomy, 175
true leg length, 38–39, 177
tumors, of bone. *See* bone tumors
two-stage exchange arthroplasty, 163
Tylenol. *See* acetaminophen
Tylenol No. 3 with Codeine, 128

UHMWPE. *See* ultra high molecular
        weight polyethylene
ultra high molecular weight polyethylene
        (UHMWPE), 108
ultrasound, deep vein thrombosis
        and, 165
unipolar hip replacement, 68, 211
universal proximal femur, 69
urinary retention, catheter for, 132–133,
        188
urologic problems, pain and, 49
urologist, 133

valgus osteotomy, 82
Vancomycin, 130, 160, 163
varus osteotomy, 82
venography, deep vein thrombosis and, 165
vessels, injury to, 185–187
        causes of, 186
        surgery for, 186
        symptoms of, 186
Vicodin, 128
Virchow's triad, blood clot formation
        and, 164

walker, as assistive aid, 137–138
walking, long distance, 152
Warfarin, 134, 167

weight bearing, after total hip replacement,
        129, 137–138
weight gain, mobility limitation and, 4
weight loss, arthritis and, 52–53
white blood cell count, infection and,
        157, 161
working, after total hip replacement,
        148–149
wound care, after total hip replacement, 141
wound debridement, infection and, 159
wound hematoma, 156
wrong site surgery, hip replacement and,
        223–224

x-ray(s), 37, 42–44
        avascular necrosis and, 22
        of bipolar hip replacement, 72
        bone spurs on, 44
        bone tumors on, 44
        bone-on-bone on, 14, 15, 43
        component loosening and, 192, 193, 194,
            195, 196
        deformities on, 43
        heterotopic ossification and, 181
        of hip fusion, 78
        hyaline cartilage on, 43
        infection and, 158
        protrusio on, 44
        sclerosis on, 43
        as template, 44
        trabecular pattern on, 43
        views of, 42–43

YOC. *See* Your Orthopaedic Connection
Your Orthopaedic Connection (YOC), 232

zirconia, 122